Series editor
Daniel Horton-Szar
BSc (Hons)
United Medical and Dental
Schools of Guy's and
St Thomas's Hospitals
(UMDS),
London

Faculty advisor
David B Jones
PhD
Reader in Pathology
University of Southampton

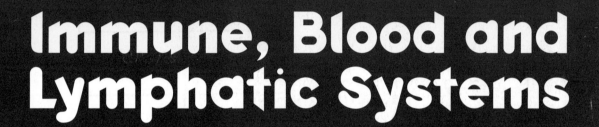

Immune, Blood and Lymphatic Systems

Saimah Arif
BSc (Hons)
United Medical and
Dental Schools of Guy's
and St Thomas's
Hospitals (UMDS),
London

Arjmand Mufti
BSc (Hons)
United Medical and
Dental Schools of Guy's
and St Thomas's
Hospitals (UMDS),
London

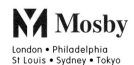 Mosby

London • Philadelphia
St Louis • Sydney • Tokyo

Editor	Louise Crowe
Development Editors	Filipa Maia
	Michele Campbell
Project Manager	Linda Horrell
Designer	Greg Smith
Layout	Paul Phillips
Illustration Management	Danny Pyne
Illustrators	Paul Bernson
	Deborah Gyan
	Jenni Miller
	Mike Saiz
	Gisli Thor
Cover Design	Greg Smith
Production	Gudrun Hughes
Index	Janine Ross

ISBN 0 7234 2993 6

Copyright © Mosby International Ltd, 1998.

Published by Mosby, an imprint of Mosby International Ltd, Lynton House, 7–12 Tavistock Square, London WC1H 9LB, UK.

Printed in Barcelona, Spain, by Grafos S.A. Arte sobre papel, 1998.
Text set in Crash Course–VAG Light; captions in Crash Course–VAG Thin.

Every effort has been made to contact holders of copyright to obtain permission to reproduce copyright material. However, if any have been inadvertently overlooked, the publishers will be pleased to make the necessary arrangements at the first opportunity.

The publisher, author and faculty advisor have undertaken reasonable endeavours to check drugs, dosages, adverse effects and contraindications in this book. We recommend that the reader should always check the manufacturer's instructions and information in the British National Formulary (BNF) or similar publication before administering any drug.

Cataloguing in Publication Data
Catalogue records for this book are available from the British Library.

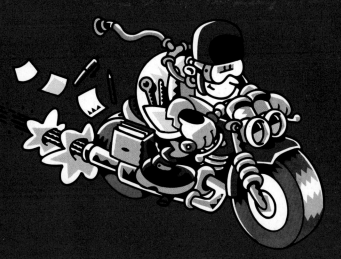

Immune, Blood and Lymphatic Systems

Preface

Immunology is a subject that many medical students find hard to master because of its conceptual nature. Haematology, for the medical student, is factual rather than conceptual, and the main problem is one of sifting through a large volume of information.

In this book, we have tried to present the information in a clear and concise manner, emphasizing points of particular importance to medical students (and to examiners!). The clinical aspects of these subjects are presented alongside the basic sciences so that the student can appreciate the link between the two, facilitating greater understanding and easier learning.

Enjoy!

Saimah Arif
Arjmand Mufti

Immunology, as with many areas of medicine, is a constantly evolving science. Nevertheless, the authors of this book have endeavoured to present all the relevant information relating to the current medical curriculum as recommended by the General Medical Council.

This volume fulfils the need to supply a revision text that covers the essential aspects of the normal physiology and pathology of the lymphoreticular system. The aim throughout has been to provide a concise and readable text with clearly drawn and easy-to-understand illustrations. In addition, hints and tips boxes and comprehension check boxes aid learning and understanding. At the end of the book there is a practice exam for self-assessment.

We hope that Crash Course Immune, Blood, and Lymphatic Systems will provide useful revision material which is relevant to the current revised medical curricula.

David Jones
Faculty Advisor

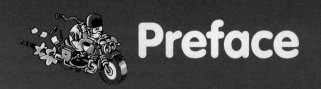

Preface

OK, no-one ever said medicine was going to be easy, but the thing is, there are very few parts of this enormous subject that are actually difficult to understand. The problem for most of us is the sheer volume of information that must be absorbed before each round of exams. It's not fun when time is getting short and you realize that: a) you really should have done a bit more work by now; and b) there are large gaps in your lecture notes that you meant to copy up but never quite got round to.

This series has been designed and written by senior medical students and doctors with recent experience of basic medical science exams. We've brought together all the information you need into compact, manageable volumes that integrate basic science with clinical skills. There is a consistent structure and layout across the series, and every title is checked for accuracy by senior faculty members from medical schools across the UK.

I hope this book makes things a little easier!

Danny Horton-Szar
Series Editor (Basic Medical Sciences)

Acknowledgements

We would like to thank Professor Bill Noble, Dr Sue Howell, Dr Graham Wallace, Robin Wolstencroft and Brian Ellis for encouraging and fostering our interest in Immunology; Clare Tibbatts for her help in the typing of the manuscripts and all of the team at Mosby for their help and advice whilst writing the book.

Figure Credits

Figures 2.1, 2.2, 2.3, 2.4, 3.1, 3.7, 3.8, 3.9, 3.15, 3.17, 3.23, 3.26, 3.28, 4.8, 12.1 and 12.10 taken from *Immunology 4e*, by I Roitt, D Male and J Brostoff, TMIP, 1996.

Figure 3.3 taken from *Advanced Immunology 3e*, by D Male, TMIP, 1996.

Figures 4.7, 5.12, and 6.1a taken from *Human Histology 2e*, by A Stevens and J Lowe, TMIP, 1997.

Figure 5.1 taken from *Human Histology 2e*, by A. Stevens and J. Lowe, TMIP, 1997. Courtesy of Trevor Gray.

Figures 6.3, 11.12, 11.13, 11.14, 11.15, 11.16, 11.17, 11.18, 11.19, 11.20, 11.21, 11.22, 11.23, 11.24 and 11.25 taken from *Clinical Haematology 2e*, TMIP, 1994. Courtesy of I Hoffbrand and J Petit.

Figures 11.26 and 11.27 taken from *Blood in Systemic Disease*, Mosby, 1997. Courtesy of M. Makris and M. Greaves. .

Contents

Preface   iii
Acknowledgements   v
Dedication   viii

Part I: Development, Structure and Function   **1**

1. Overview of the Immune , Blood and Lymphatic Systems   **3**
The players–an overview of the cell lines   3

2. Organization of the Lymphoid System   **7**
Primary lymphoid organs   7
Secondary lymphoid organs   9

3. Concepts of Immunity   **15**
Innate and adaptive immunity   15
The innate immune system   16
Recognition molecules: The B cell   22
Recognition molecules: The T cell   26
Generation of antigen receptor diversity   30
Humoral immunity   33
Cell-mediated immunity   35
The complement system   38

4. The Immune System in Disease   **43**
Response to tissue damage   43
Hypersensitivity mechanisms   49
Immune response to pathogens   51
Autoimmunity and immune disease   53
Immunization   55
Transplantation   58

5. Red Blood Cells and Haemoglobin   **61**
Structure and function of erythrocytes   61
Erythropoiesis   63
Iron and haem metabolism   65
Haemoglobin   68
The red cell cytoskeleton   72
Metabolism of red cells   73

6. Haemostasis   **77**
Platelets and blood coagulation   77
The coagulation cascade   80

7. Serum Proteins   **85**
Normal serum proteins   85
Acute phase proteins   87

8. Serology and Blood Transfusion   **89**
Red cell antigens   89
Blood transfusion   91

Part II: Clinical Assessment	**93**
9. Taking a History	**95**
Structure of a history	95
Common presenting complaints	97
10. Clinical Examination	**101**
11. Further Investigations	**105**
Haematological investigations	105
Investigation of immune Function	110
Part III: Basic Pathology	**119**
12. Disorders of Immunity	**121**
Autoimmune disease	121
Diseases of immune deficiency	124
Amyloidosis	130
13. Disorders of White Cells, Lymph Nodes and the Spleen	**133**
Leukopenia	133
Reactive proliferation of white cells	134
Neoplastic proliferation of white cells	134
Disorders of the spleen	143
14. Disorders of Red Cells	**145**
Anaemia due to blood loss	145
Anaemia due to red cell destruction (haemolytic anaemias)	146
Anaemia due to impaired red cell production	152
15. Disorders of Red Cells	**155**
Bleeding disorders : platelets	155
Bleeding disorders : clotting factor abnormalities	158
Thrombosis	159
Part IV: Self-assessment	**161**
Multiple-choice questions	163
Short-answer questions	168
Essay questions	169
MCQ answers	170
SAQ answers	171
Index	**175**

To my family   SA

To my family and in memory of Abba-jaan   AM

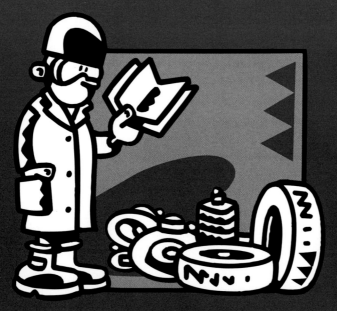

DEVELOPMENT, STRUCTURE, AND FUNCTION

1. Overview of the Immune, Blood, and Lymphatic Systems   3

2. Organization of the Lymphoid System   7

3. Concepts of Immunity   15

4. The Immune System in Disease   43

5. Red Blood Cells and Haemoglobin   61

6. Haemostasis   77

7. Serum Proteins   85

8. Serology and Blood Transfusion   89

1. Overview of the Immune, Blood, and Lymphatic Systems

THE PLAYERS—AN OVERVIEW OF THE CELL LINES

All mature blood cells are derived from a common stem cell. Haemopoiesis is the formation and development of red and white blood cells from these undifferentiated stem cells. Haemopoietic stem cells are pluripotent, i.e. they are capable of differentiating along a number of pathways and have an unlimited capacity for self-renewal, thus maintaining a reserve population.

Stem cells yield one of three main cell lineages:
- Erythroid → erythrocytes.
- Lymphoid → lymphocytes.
- Myeloid → neutrophils, basophils, eosinophils, monocytes, and megakaryocytes.

Subsequent differentiation of the erythroid, lymphoid, and myeloid cells gives rise to specialized progenitor cells for each type of mature blood cell. These cells are not capable of self-renewal (Fig. 1.1).

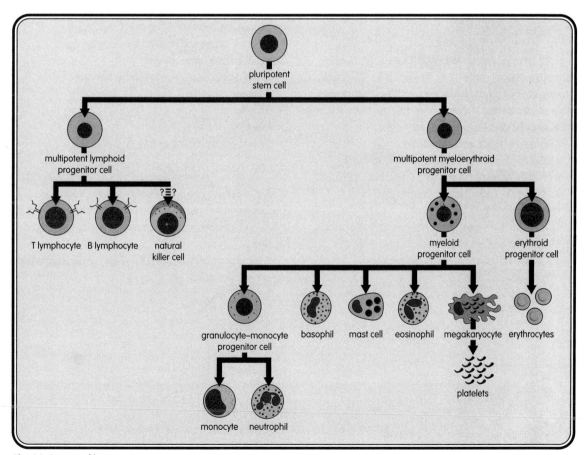

Fig. 1.1 Stages of haemopoiesis.

Sites of haemopoiesis

The site of haemopoiesis changes according to developmental age:

- Birth to 6 weeks—fetal yolk sac.
- From 6 weeks to 6 months—fetal liver.
- From 6 months onwards—bone marrow.

Myeloid cells

The first progenitor cell produced when haemopoietic stem cells are grown *in vitro* is the colony-forming unit (CFU). This is capable of giving rise to granulocytes, erythrocytes, monocytes, and megakaryocytes (CFU-GEMM). Various growth factors, or cytokines, are required for the proliferation and differentiation of haemopoietic cells, including colony-stimulating factors (CSFs). Major CSFs that have been identified include:

- Multilineage CSF (also known as interleukin-3).
- Granulocyte–macrophage CSF (GM-CSF).
- Macrophage CSF (M-CSF).
- Granulocyte CSF (G-CSF).

A group of cytokines called interleukins (ILs) are also involved in the regulation of haemopoiesis. They are produced primarily by the bone marrow stromal cells. Stem cell factor (SCF), also secreted by the bone marrow stromal cells, acts on primitive stem cells.

CSFs act in a sequential manner:

1. Multi-CSF acts early in differentiation, to induce formation of all non-lymphoid blood cells including erythrocytes, granulocytes, monocytes, and megakaryocytes.
2. GM-CSF acts on the same cell lines at a later stage.
3. M-CSF and G-CSF act later still, to stimulate the formation of monocytes and neutrophils, respectively.

Specific cytokine receptors are expressed on the membrane of each progenitor cell and are pivotal in subsequent differentiation and maturation, e.g. the macrophage progenitor cell expresses specific receptors for M-CSF, the binding of which stimulates cellular proliferation and differentiation.

Erythropoietin, a haemopoietic cytokine, is produced by the kidney. It is involved in terminal erythrocyte development and regulates red blood cell production.

Lymphoid cells

Lymphoid progenitor cells differentiate to form three distinct cell types:

- B cell.
- T cell.
- Natural killer (NK) cell.

Lymphocytes comprise 20–40% of the body's white blood cells. They circulate in the blood and lymph, and also have the capacity to migrate into tissue spaces and lymphoid organs. The B cell receptor is a membrane-bound antibody molecule; the T cell expresses the T cell receptor.

B and T cells share the following features:

- Diversity.
- Specificity.
- Memory.
- Discrimination between self and non-self.

NK cells do not express antigenic receptors and hence do not express specificity. However, they have been implicated in tumour lysis and protection against viral infections, although the exact mechanisms remain unclear.

A general overview of the functions of different blood cells is shown in Fig. 1.2.

- **Describe the concepts underlying haemopoiesis.**
- **What are the processes via which myeloid and lymphoid cells are produced?**
- **Summarize the functions of blood cells.**

Blood cell functions	
Cell type	**Functions**
erythrocytes	carry O_2 from lungs to tissues, and CO_2 from tissues to lungs
neutrophils	usually first to arrive at point of inflammation by chemotaxis—phagocytosis and the killing of phagocytosed bacteria
basophils	non-phagocytic—major role in allergic responses via release of mediators, e.g. histamine; may also play role in immunity against parasites
eosinophils	as for neutrophils, although decreased phagocytic function; play major role in defence against parasites; dampen inflammatory response in immediate-type hypersensitivity via release of histaminase and aryl sulphatase, which inactivate mast cell products such as histamine
monocytes	phagocytosis and removal of antigen; act as antigen-presenting cells (APCs)
platelets	adhere to exposed subendothelial connective tissue and participate in blood clotting
lymphocytes	key players in adaptive immune response; release haemopoietic substances

Fig. 1.2 Blood cell functions.

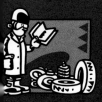

2. Organization of the Lymphoid System

Lymphoid organs and tissues are classified as primary (central) or secondary (peripheral).

PRIMARY LYMPHOID ORGANS

The bone marrow and thymus comprise the primary lymphoid organs and are the main sites of lymphocyte development and maturation.

Bone marrow

Haemopoietic tissue fills all of the bone cavities in the newborn, but in the adult, haemopoiesis is restricted principally to the sternum, vertebrae, pelvis, and ribs. The total volume of haemopoietic tissue is 1–2 litres. Because of its macroscopic appearance, this tissue is known as red marrow. Approximately 50% of red marrow consists of fat. The marrow in the peripheral skeleton—yellow marrow—contains mainly fat. However, yellow marrow still contains a small population of precursor cells that may be reactivated when the demand for blood cells is sufficiently high. Similarly, the liver and spleen can resume their fetal haemopoietic role if required.

The red marrow provides a suitable micro-environment for stem cell growth and development. It has two main components:

- Specialized fibroblasts, known as adventitial reticular cells, which secrete a framework of reticulin fibres (fine collagen fibres), forming a meshwork that plays an essential role in supporting the developing blood cells.
- A network of blood sinusoids, lined by a single layer of endothelial cells, which interconnect via tight junctions and thus effectively separate the vascular and extravascular spaces.

The nutrient artery of the bone marrow branches into a network of vascular sinuses that support the haemopoietic cells. These drain into a large central sinus that channels the blood into the systemic venous circulation. Haemopoiesis takes place in haemopoietic cords or islands located between the vascular sinuses.

Macrophages are found within the haemopoietic cords at the centre of each focal group and contain stored iron in the form of ferritin and haemosiderin. They have three main functions:

- Transfer of iron to developing erythroblasts for haemoglobin synthesis.
- Phagocytosis of the cellular debris of haemopoiesis.
- Regulation of haemopoietic cell differentiation and maturation.

Newly formed cells from the haemopoietic system enter the bloodstream in areas where the endothelial cell cytoplasm lining the sinusoids thins to approaching a double plasma membrane in thickness.

The thymus

T cell progenitors enter the thymus gland as immature thymocytes and emerge as mature, antigen-specific, immunocompetent T cells. The thymus is a bilobed

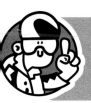

In humans, B cells mature in the bone marrow, and T cells in the thymus. (B cells acquire their title from their site of development in birds—the bursa of Fabricius.)

gland located in the anterior part of the superior mediastinum, posterior to the sternum and anterior to the great vessels and upper part of the heart. It may extend superiorly into the roof of the neck and inferiorly into the anterior mediastinum. Each lobe is surrounded by a capsule and divided into multiple lobules by fibrous septa known as trabeculae. Each lobule is divided into two regions (Fig. 2.1):
* An outer cortex.
* An inner medulla.

It is thought that T cells enter the thymus via the cortex, where they rapidly proliferate. The thymus exhibits a high rate of cell death, and a much smaller and more mature group of thymocytes survives to enter the medulla. The thymocytes continue to mature here and eventually leave the thymus via the postcapillary venules.

A network of epithelial cells is present in the thymic lobules:

* The 'nurse' cells of the outer cortex.
* The cortical epithelial cells.
* The medullary epithelial cells.

These are all vital in the development of thymocytes into mature T cells. A 'nurse' cell is capable of engulfing up to 50 thymocytes with its long membranous processes. Cortical epithelial cells have long, interconnecting, cytoplasmic processes that interact with thymocytes. In addition, bone-marrow-derived interdigitating (ID) cells and macrophages are present, especially at the corticomedullary junction, and they also have long processes that interact with thymocytes. Collectively, these cells are known as stromal cells.

Thymic epithelial cells produce hormones that are essential for the differentiation and maturation of thymocytes. Four hormones have been isolated so far:
* α thymosin.
* β_4 thymosin.
* Thymulin.
* Thymopoietin.

Fig. 2.1 Ultrastructure of the thymus, showing the cells present in the cortex and medulla.

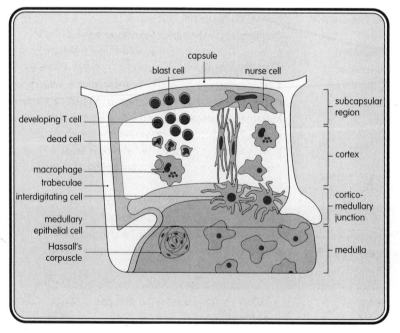

Only 1–5% of thymocytes in the thymus reach maturity, the remainder undergoing programmed cell death (apoptosis).

Hassall's corpuscles are structures containing degenerating epithelial cells, found in the thymic medulla. Their exact function is unclear.

The human embryonic thymus develops from the third pharyngeal pouch during week 4 or 5 of gestation. Dorsally, the pharyngeal pouch differentiates into the inferior parathyroid glands, and the elongated ventral portions fuse to form the bilobed thymus gland by week 8. Both the thymus and the parathyroid glands migrate inferiorly and later separate.

Developmental timescale
Cell development within the thymus occurs as follows:
- Week 10: 95% of cells belong to the T cell lineage; a few erythroblasts and Hassall's corpuscles are also present.
- Week 14: interdigitating cells and macrophages appear.
- Week 17: the thymus is fully differentiated and producing viable-lymphocytes.

Although it continues to grow until puberty, the relative size of the thymus gland decreases over this period. After puberty, there is a real reduction in size, and by adulthood, it is composed largely of adipose tissue. However, it continues to produce T lymphocytes.

In DiGeorge syndrome, the thymus fails to develop. Consequently, there is an absence of circulating T cells and a reduction in cell-mediated immunity.

- Describe the structure and function of the bone marrow and thymus.
- Summarize the embryology of the thymus.
- What is DiGeorge syndrome?

SECONDARY LYMPHOID ORGANS

The lymph nodes, spleen, and mucosal associated lymphoid tissue (MALT) constitute the secondary lymphoid organs. They provide a site for lymphocytes to interact with antigen and other cells of the immune system.

Lymphatic drainage and lymph nodes
The relatively high hydrostatic pressure of blood at the arterial end of capillaries exceeds the osmotic pressure of plasma proteins, causing water and low-molecular-weight solutes to leak out into tissue spaces. This is known as interstitial fluid. Most of the fluid returns to the venous circulation as the pressure gradient is reversed at the venous end.

The lymphatic system provides an additional route for the return of this fluid from the interstitial spaces to the blood. Once it has entered a lymphatic vessel, interstitial fluid is known as lymph. Lymphatic vessels are present in all tissues and organs of the body except for the following:
- CNS.
- Cornea.
- Internal ear.
- Epidermis of the skin.
- Cartilage.
- Bone marrow.

Lymphatic circulation
Lymph nodes are present throughout the lymphatic system, often occurring at junctions of the lymphatic vessels. Several afferent vessels carry lymph into the lymph nodes, and one efferent vessel drains it off. Lymph vessels contain numerous valves that are important in preventing back-flow of lymph. The lymphatic system is not circulatory, i.e. lymph is not pumped around the body, but acts as a passive drainage system, returning interstitial fluid to the bloodstream.

Lymph nodes act as filters, 'sampling' lymphatic fluid on its way to the systemic circulation for bacteria, viruses, and foreign particles. They frequently form chains, and may drain a specific organ or area of the body. For example:
- Cervical lymph nodes drain the head and neck.
- Axillary lymph nodes drain the upper limb and areas of the trunk.

- Inguinal lymph nodes drain the lower limb.
- Abdominal nodes drain the abdomen.
- Superior and inferior mesenteric lymph nodes drain the alimentary canal.

Lymph returns to the circulation at lymphovenous junctions. On the right side, lymph passes via the right lymphatic duct and empties into the venous system at the junction of the right subclavian vein and right internal jugular vein. This system provides drainage for:
- The right half of the head and neck.
- The right side of the thorax.
- The right arm.
- The trunk down to the umbilicus.

On the left side, lymph passes via the thoracic duct and empties into the venous system at the junction of the left subclavian vein and left internal jugular vein. This provides drainage for:

- The left half of the head and neck.
- The lower part of body.
- The left arm.
- The left side of the thorax.

Accessory lymphatic vessels, which join with the venous circulation at the same locations, drain the rest of the body.

Lymph node structure

Lymph nodes can be divided into three areas (Fig. 2.2):
- Cortex.
- Paracortex.
- Central medulla.

Cortex

The cortex contains mainly B cells, initially organized as primary follicles. When stimulated by antigen, primary follicles form secondary follicles, each containing a germinal centre.

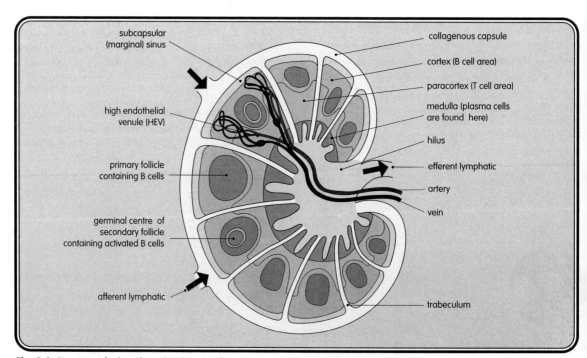

Fig. 2.2 Structure of a lymph node, showing the cortex, paracortex, and medulla.

Paracortex
The paracortex contains T cells and dendritic cells that are antigen-presenting cells (APCs). The latter express high levels of class II MHC molecules, which are essential for antigen presentation to T helper (Th) cells.

Medulla
The medulla contains cellular cords that are sparsely populated with B and T lymphocytes, plasma cells, and macrophages. The cords are located around medullary sinuses. The lymph drains into a terminal sinus, which eventually forms the efferent lymphatic vessel.

Lymphatic flow in lymph nodes
Lymph flows into lymph nodes via several afferent vessels which empty into the subcapsular sinus. It percolates through the cortex, paracortex, and medulla. If foreign macromolecules—e.g. bacteria or particulate

matter—are present, activation of B and T cells occurs (see Chapter 3).

There is a greater number of lymphocytes in the efferent vessels compared with the afferent ones because:
* Antigenic challenge results in stimulation and proliferation of lymphocytes.
* Blood-borne lymphocytes enter the lymph node via specialized high endothelial venules (HEVs) in the paracortex.

Lymphocyte recirculation refers to the continuous movement of lymphocytes through blood and lymph, which is essential for a normal immune response (Fig. 2.3). Approximately 1–2% of the lymphocytic pool recirculates each hour. This increases the chances of an antigenically committed lymphocyte encountering complementary antigen in the peripheral lymphoid organs.

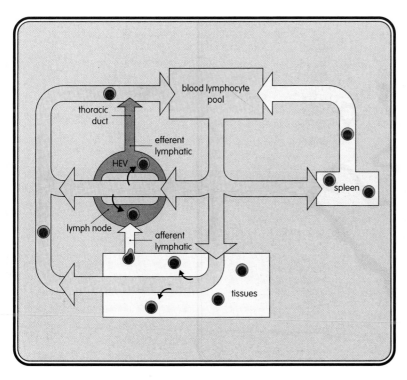

Fig. 2.3 Lymphocyte recirculation. Lymphocytes enter lymph nodes directly from the systemic circulation via specialized high endothelial venules (HEVs). Afferent lymphatics also carry lymphocytes to the lymph nodes. Lymphocytes leave lymph nodes via efferent lymphatics, and rejoin the systemic venous circulation via the right lymphatic duct or the thoracic duct.

The spleen

The spleen is derived from the primitive gut and first appears in week 5 of fetal development. Unlike the lymph nodes, the spleen has no afferent lymphatics. It is specialized for filtering blood much as the lymph nodes filter lymph. It therefore provides a capacity for responding to systemic infections. It is surrounded by a capsule of collagenous fibres that penetrate into the organ and are known as trabeculae.

The relations of the spleen comprise:

- Anterior—the stomach, tail of the pancreas, and left colic flexure.
- Medial—the left kidney.
- Posterior—the diaphragm, left pleura, left lung, and ribs 9–11.

Blood supply to the spleen is via the splenic artery. Blood is drained via the splenic veins, which join the superior mesenteric vein to form the portal vein.

The two main types of tissues found within the spleen are red pulp and white pulp. These are separated by a marginal zone (Fig. 2.4). The red pulp consists of a network of sinusoids containing macrophages, erythrocytes, platelets, granulocytes, lymphocytes, and plasma cells. The removal and destruction of aged and defective erythrocytes and platelets by macrophages takes place here. Blood cells not removed can re-enter the blood circulation. The splenic white pulp consists of lymphoid tissue. The periarteriolar lymphoid sheath (PALS), which predominantly contains T cells, surrounds the central arteriole. B cells are arranged into follicles that may be primary (unstimulated) but will be secondary in most patients.

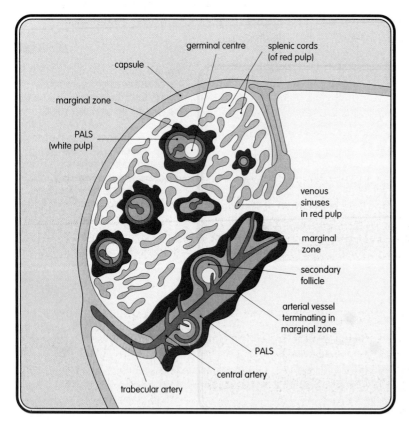

Fig. 2.4 Organization of lymphoid tissue in the spleen.

Lymphocytes enter the spleen via the marginal zone and migrate to their respective B and T cell domains. Splenic macrophages enter the spleen as monocytes. As well as having immunological functions, the spleen acts as a reservoir for platelets, erythrocytes, and granulocytes.

Mucosal associated lymphoid tissue

This consists of unencapsulated subepithelial lymphoid tissue found in the gastrointestinal, respiratory, and urogenital tracts. Mucosal associated lymphoid tissue (MALT) can be subdivided into:

- Organized lymphoid tissue, e.g. tonsils, appendix, Peyer's patches.
- Diffuse lymphoid tissue located in the lamina propria of intestinal villi and lungs.

Organized lymphoid tissue

Tonsils

The lingual, palatine, and nasopharyngeal tonsils contain many germinating centres and protect against antigen entering via the oronasal route.

Respiratory tract

Lymphoid tissues in the bronchi contain dendritic cells that act as APCs and process and present antigen.

Gastrointestinal tract

Peyer's patches are organized submucosal lymphoid follicles present throughout the large and small intestine, being particularly prominent in the lower ileum.

The epithelium above Peyer's patches consists of specialized M cells that sample the lumen of the gut for antigen, endocytose it, and may present it to subepithelial lymphoid cells. This results in the stimulation of B cells, which move out of the follicles and 'home' to diffuse MALT, where they differentiate into plasma cells and secrete IgA antibody. IgA is released onto the abluminal surface and binds the poly-IgA receptor on epithelial cells. The receptor–antibody complex is endocytosed and transported across the cell to the luminal surface and released into the gut lumen.

Lymphocyte trafficking in MALT

Mucosal lymphocytes generally recirculate within the mucosal lymphoid system. This is facilitated by interactions between specific adhesion molecules expressed on the surfaces of lymphocytes derived from Peyer's patches and corresponding ligands present on the venular endothelium.

A common exam question is: 'Write about the primary and secondary lymphoid organs'. The student must know both these topics very well and there should be no confusion between the classifications.

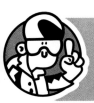

- Describe the structure and function of the lymph nodes and spleen.
- Describe lymphocyte recirculation.
- Summarize the structure of MALT and explain how lymphocytes recirculate within the mucosal lymphoid system.

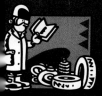

3. Concepts of Immunity

INNATE AND ADAPTIVE IMMUNITY

Immunity is a state of relative resistance to disease.

Innate immunity involves inherent non-specific mechanisms that are not altered upon repeated exposure to antigen.

Adaptive immunity is characterized by:
- Specificity—the ability of the adaptive immune response to distinguish differences between antigens.
- Memory—the fact that once the adaptive immune system has responded to an antigen (the primary response), it responds more rapidly and to a greater degree upon subsequent exposures (the secondary response; Fig. 3.1).

Compared with the primary antibody response, the secondary antibody response is characterized by:
- Higher antibody titres.
- Peak antibody levels that are attained sooner and persist for longer.
- Higher affinity for antigen.
- Production of mainly IgG and relatively low IgM levels in the circulation.

Some important definitions are:
- **Antigen**—any molecule that can be recognized by the adaptive immune system.
- **Immunogen**—a molecule that evokes an immune response. All immunogens are antigenic, but not all antigens are immunogenic.
- **Hapten**—a small antigen that is not immunogenic unless coupled to a larger carrier molecule.
- **Epitope** (antigenic determinant)—the discrete area of the antigen that is recognized by the adaptive immune response. A single antigen may have several different epitopes, each of which is recognized by a different antibody or T cell receptor (TCR).
- **Cytokines**—secreted, low-molecular-weight proteins that act locally by binding specific receptors on target cells.

The innate and adaptive immune systems comprise both cellular and secreted components (Fig. 3.2).

Fig. 3.1 Primary and secondary antibody responses.

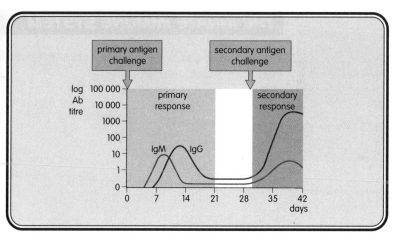

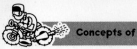

Components of the innate and adaptive immune systems		
	Innate	**Adaptive**
cellular components	monocytes	B cells and plasma cells
	macrophages	T cells
	neutrophils	antigen-presenting cells (APCs)
	eosinophils	
	basophils	
	mast cells	
	natural killer (NK) cells	
secreted factors	complement	antibody
	cytokines	complement
	lysozyme	cytokines
	acute phase proteins	
	interferons	

Fig. 3.2 Components of the innate and adaptive immune systems.

 Primary and secondary antibody responses illustrate adaptive immunity – a basic immunological concept that often crops up in exams. So make sure you can sketch Fig. 3.1 and you can discuss the differences between the primary and secondary antibody responses.

○ What are the differences between innate and adaptive immunity?
○ Define the terms antigen, immunogen, hapten, epitope, and cytokine.

THE INNATE IMMUNE SYSTEM

Innate defences against infection can be classified into three main groups:
- Skin and mucosal membranes.
- Soluble proteins.
- Cellular components.

Skin and mucosal membranes

Skin and mucosal membranes act as physical barriers to the entry of pathogens. Sebaceous glands produce sebum that has a high fatty acid and lactic acid content, maintaining the skin pH between 3 and 5 and inhibiting the growth of microorganisms. Mucosal membranes are protected by various factors:

- The flushing action of saliva, tears, and urine.
- Mucus secreted by the epithelium of the lower respiratory tract, which entraps microorganisms and is propelled upwards by beating cilia (mucociliary escalator).

Both the skin and the mucosal membranes are protected by the normal microflora of the human body. However, if this is disrupted by the use of antibiotics, the growth of pathogenic organisms may be unrestricted. Other factors inhibiting the growth of pathogens include body temperature, high O_2 tension (e.g. in the lungs), and acidic pH (e.g. in the vagina and stomach).

Soluble proteins

The soluble proteins that contribute to innate immunity are listed in Fig. 3.3.

Cells of innate immunity
Granulocytes

The term granulocyte encompasses neutrophils, basophils and eosinophils (Fig. 3.4). Granulocytes are characterized by a highly granulated cytoplasm and polymorphic nuclei (are therefore also called polymorphonuclear cells, although this tends to be used interchangeably with 'neutrophils' as these make up the vast majority of the granulocytes).

Neutrophils

Neutrophils (see Fig. 3.4) comprise 50–70% of circulating white cells. They circulate in blood for 7–10 hours and then migrate to the tissues, where they have a lifespan of 1–3 days. They are the first cells to arrive at the site of inflammation, and their primary function is phagocytosis. Defunct neutrophils are the major constituent of pus.

Soluble proteins contributing to innate immunity	
Protein	**Notes**
lysozyme	bactericidal enzyme in mucus, saliva, tears, sweat and breast milk; cleaves peptidoglycan layer of bacterial cell wall
interferons	family of proteins secreted by virus-infected cells; induce antiviral state in neighbouring, uninfected cells
complement	group of ~20 serum proteins, proenzymes; activation leads to enzyme cascade, the products of which enhance phagocytosis and mediate cell lysis; alternative pathway can be activated by non-specific mechanisms
lactoferrin	iron-binding protein that competes with microorganisms for iron, an essential metabolite
C-reactive protein	acute phase protein, synthesized in liver; serum concentration rises >100-fold in tissue-damaging infections; binds C-polysaccharide cell wall component of bacteria and fungi; activates complement via classical pathway; acts as opsonin, enhancing phagocytosis

Fig. 3.3 Some of the major soluble proteins contributing to innate immunity.

Fig. 3.4 Structure of granulocytes.

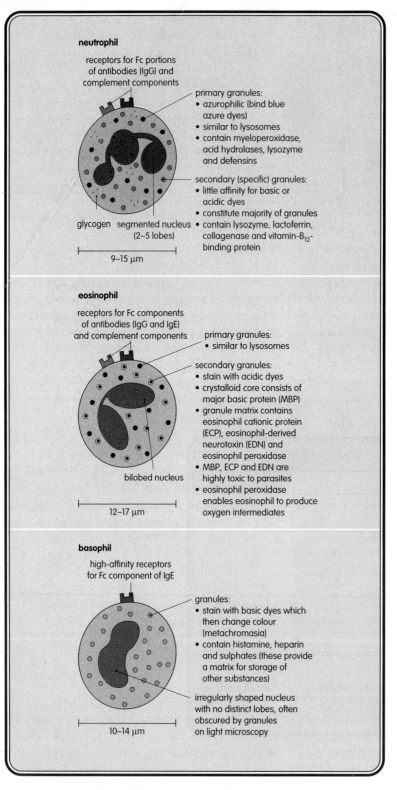

neutrophil

receptors for Fc portions
of antibodies (IgG) and
complement components

primary granules:
- azurophilic (bind blue
  azure dyes)
- similar to lysosomes
- contain myeloperoxidase,
  acid hydrolases, lysozyme
  and defensins

secondary (specific) granules:
- little affinity for basic or
  acidic dyes
- constitute majority of granules
- contain lysozyme, lactoferrin,
  collagenase and vitamin-B_{12}-
  binding protein

glycogen   segmented nucleus
(2–5 lobes)

9–15 μm

eosinophil

receptors for Fc components
of antibodies (IgG and IgE)
and complement components

primary granules:
- similar to lysosomes

secondary granules:
- stain with acidic dyes
- crystalloid core consists of
  major basic protein (MBP)
- granule matrix contains
  eosinophil cationic protein
  (ECP), eosinophil-derived
  neurotoxin (EDN) and
  eosinophil peroxidase
- MBP, ECP and EDN are
  highly toxic to parasites
- eosinophil peroxidase
  enables eosinophil to produce
  oxygen intermediates

bilobed nucleus

12–17 μm

basophil

high-affinity receptors
for Fc component of IgE

granules:
- stain with basic dyes which
  then change colour
  (metachromasia)
- contain histamine, heparin
  and sulphates (these provide
  a matrix for storage of
  other substances)

irregularly shaped nucleus
with no distinct lobes, often
obscured by granules
on light microscopy

10–14 μm

• **Oxygen-independent degradation**—by lysozyme, lactoferrin, hydrolytic enzymes, and defensins, contained within the neutrophil granules; they do not require oxygen for their action.

• **Oxygen-dependent degradation**—during phagocytosis, oxidases in neutrophil granules catalyse the reduction of oxygen to a superoxide radical ($O_2^{\cdot-}$), from which other oxidizing agents such as the hydroxyl radical ($OH\cdot$) and hydrogen peroxide (H_2O_2) are generated. Hydrogen peroxide combines with chloride ions to form hypochlorous acid ($HOCl$) in a reaction catalysed by myeloperoxidase, an enzyme found in neutrophilic primary granules. Hypochlorous acid reacts with amines to produce chloramines ($R\text{-}NCl$). $HOCl$ and $R\text{-}NCl$ are longer-lived than the other oxidizing agents and are probably the most important compounds in target killing *in vivo*. The formation of oxygen intermediates is accompanied by a pronounced respiratory burst.

If a target cannot be easily phagocytosed, the neutrophil may release its granule contents extracellularly, causing tissue damage.

Eosinophils

Eosinophils (see Fig. 3.4) comprise 1–3% of circulating white cells and are found principally in tissues (stay in blood for less than 1 hour). They are capable of phagocytosis, but this is not their primary function. They are important in defence against parasites and cause damage by extracellular degranulation. Their products are anti-inflammatory and can inactivate mast cell products. They are derived from CFU-Eo and their maturation is the same as for the neutrophil, i.e. myeloblast → promyelocyte → myelocyte → metamyelocyte → mature granulocyte. IL-5 is an important eosinophil growth factor.

Basophils

Basophils (see Fig. 3.4) comprise <1% of circulating white cells. They function by discharging their granule contents and are important in allergic responses (type I hypersensitivity reactions), where they play a similar role to mast cells. They are derived from CFU-B and they mature by the same stages as neutrophils.

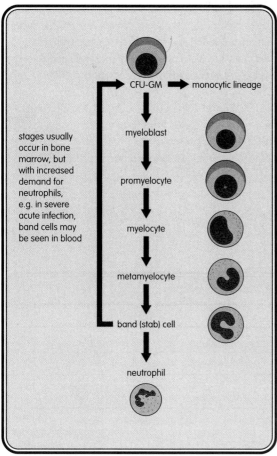

Fig. 3.5 Production of neutrophils.

stages usually occur in bone marrow, but with increased demand for neutrophils, e.g. in severe acute infection, band cells may be seen in blood

CFU-GM → monocytic lineage
myeloblast
promyelocyte
myelocyte
metamyelocyte
band (stab) cell
neutrophil

During cell differentiation (Fig. 3.5), the following changes occur:
• Increased segmentation of the nucleus.
• Loss of rough endoplasmic reticulum and Golgi apparatus.
• Appearance of characteristic cytoplasmic granules.

In response to tissue damage, neutrophils will migrate from the bloodstream to the site of the insult (see Chapter 4). Upon contact with its target, the neutrophil extends its pseudopodia and encloses the material in a phagosome. The phagosome fuses with both primary and secondary granules, and its contents are degraded by the following pathways:

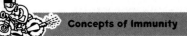

Mast cells

Mast cells are functionally similar to basophils, but are resident in the tissues. High concentrations are found close to blood vessels in connective tissue, skin, and mucosal membranes. There are two types of mast cell:

- Mucosal mast cell.
- Connective tissue mast cell.

They differ in their tissue distribution and protease content. Both mast cells and basophils have high-affinity receptors for the Fc portion of IgE. Cross-linking of these receptors results in influx of calcium ions into the cell, which induces degranulation and release of pharmacologically active mediators (Fig. 3.6). Populations of mast cells in different anatomical sites exhibit different secretory profiles.

Natural killer (NK) cells

These are also called large granular lymphocytes (LGLs) and comprise 5–10% of circulating lymphocytes. They have a role in killing tumour and virus-infected

Mast cell granule contents	
Mediator	**Actions**
Primary mediators	
histamine	↑ vascular permeability, vasodilatation, smooth muscle contraction
serotonin (5-HT)	↑ vascular permeability, vasodilatation, smooth muscle contraction, platelet aggregation
heparin	anticoagulant; modulates tryptase activity
eosinophil chemotactic factor (ECF-A)	chemotactic for eosinophils
neutrophil chemotactic factor (NCF-A)	chemotactic for neutrophils
proteases, e.g. tryptase, chymase	tryptase cleaves C3; chymase → ↑ mucus secretion
acid hydrolases, e.g. β-glucoronidase	degradation of extracellular matrix
Secondary mediators	
platelet-activating factor (PAF)	platelet aggregation and activation, ↑ vascular permeability, vasodilatation, chemotactic for leucocytes (especially eosinophils), activation of neutrophils
leukotrienes, e.g. LTC_4, LTD_4, and LTE_4 comprise SRS-A (slow-reacting substance of anaphylaxis)	SRS-A → vasodilatation, smooth muscle contraction, and mucus secretion; LTB_4 is chemotactic for neutrophils
prostaglandins (predominantly PGD_2)	vasodilatation, smooth muscle contraction, chemotactic for neutrophils, potentiation of other mediators (especially bradykinin and histamine)
bradykinin	↑ vascular permeability, vasodilatation, smooth muscle contraction, stimulation of pain nerve endings
cytokines	variety of actions

Fig. 3.6 Mast cell mediators and their actions. Primary mediators are preformed and stored in mast cell granules. Secondary mediators are synthesized or released following mast cell activation, when the cell membrane breaks down.

cells. Their lineage is uncertain—they possibly arise from an early T cell progenitor cell. They express no specific membrane markers. Their mechanism of killing is similar to that of cytotoxic T cells. Activation by IL-2 results in an increase in 'killing' ability—these cells are called lymphokine-activated killer (LAK) cells.

Mononuclear phagocyte system

Mononuclear phagocytes comprise the other major group of phagocytic cells. They are derived from CFU-GM: CFU-GM → monoblast → promonocyte → monocyte → macrophage.

Monocytes account for 5–10% of the white cell count and circulate in the blood for approximately 8 hours before migrating into the tissues, where they differentiate into macrophages. Some macrophages become adapted for specific functions in particular tissues, e.g. Kupffer cells in the liver, Langerhans' cells in the skin.

Macrophages are larger and longer-lived than monocytes, have greater phagocytic ability, and have a larger repertoire of lytic enzymes and secretory products. They phagocytose and destroy their targets using similar mechanisms to neutrophils. In addition, they can secrete a number of compounds extracellularly, including cytokines, complement components, and hydrolytic enzymes. Some of their products have anti-inflammatory actions.

Macrophages express a wide array of receptor molecules on their surfaces, e.g. FcγRI–III (receptors for the Fc portion of IgG, types I–III), complement receptors, and cytokine receptors. They can be activated by a variety of stimuli:
- Direct contact with target.
- Contact with components of the complement and blood coagulation pathways.
- Cytokines.

Activated macrophages are more efficient at phagocytosis, have greater secretory and microbicidal activity, and express higher levels of major histocompatibility complex (MHC) class II molecules than their resting counterparts. In addition to phagocytosis, macrophages are able to process and present antigen in association with class II MHC molecules. The rate of phagocytosis by neutrophils and macrophages can be greatly increased by opsonins such as IgG and C3b (neutrophils and macrophages have receptors for these molecules which may be bound to the antigenic surface).

In comparison to neutrophils, macrophages:
- Are longer-lived.
- Are larger (diameter 25–50 μm), enabling phagocytosis of larger targets.
- Move more slowly.
- Exhibit a less pronounced respiratory burst.
- Phagocytose more slowly.
- Retain Golgi apparatus and rough endoplasmic reticulum and can therefore synthesize new proteins, including lysosomal enzymes and secretory products.
- Secrete a variety of substances.
- Express class II MHC molecules and can act as antigen-presenting cells (APCs).

The last two activities are particularly important as they enable the macrophage to interact with lymphocytes and thus play a role in the adaptive immune response.

- **Describe the role of the skin, mucous membranes, and soluble proteins in defence against infectious organisms.**
- **Summarize the structure and function of the mononuclear phagocytes (monocytes and macrophages), granulocytes (neutrophils, eosinophils, and basophils), mast cells, and NK cells, and outline their role in immunity.**

RECOGNITION MOLECULES: THE B CELL

The B cell recognition molecules are called immunoglobulins or antibodies. Immunoglobulins are found on the B cell membrane and plasma cells secrete them. On serum electrophoresis, Igs migrate to the γ globulin region. There are five classes of immunoglobulin (Ig) in humans:

- IgG.
- IgA.
- IgM.
- IgE.
- IgD.

Structure of an immunoglobulin

We will consider IgG as a model for the structure of all Ig classes. IgG consists of two identical heavy (H) chains and two identical light (L) chains, linked by disulphide bridges. Digestion of IgG with papain produces two types of fragment (Fig. 3.7):

- Two Fab fragments, so called because they still bind antigen.
- One Fc fragment, so called because it can be crystallized.

These fragments correspond to the functional division of the IgG molecule: Fab fragments are involved in epitope binding and the Fc fragment has various accessory functions.

The light chain

The light chain has two regions:

- A variable region at the amino (N) terminus of the chain.
- A constant region at the carboxyl (C) terminus of the chain, which may be either κ (kappa) or λ (lambda). Approximately 60% of human light chains are κ and the rest are λ. Both of the light chains of a single Ig molecule are of one type only, i.e. both are κ or both are λ.

The heavy chain

Similarly, the heavy chain can be divided into variable and constant regions. The variable region comprises approximately 110 amino acids at the N terminus of the chain. The remainder of the chain is the constant region and defines class. The γ, α, μ, ϵ, and δ heavy chains correspond to IgG, IgA, IgM, IgE, and IgD, respectively. Minor changes in the sequence of the γ and α heavy chains give rise to subclasses of IgG (IgG1–IgG4) and IgA (IgA1 and IgA2), respectively.

Fig. 3.7 Simplified structure of IgG, showing results of papain digestion.

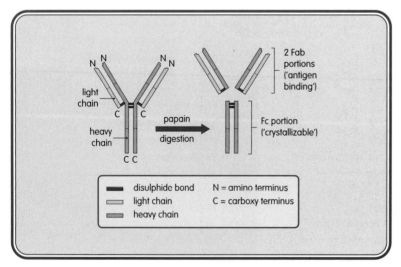

The immunoglobulin domain

Heavy and light chains are composed of motifs called domains. Each domain is approximately 110 amino acids in length and has an intrachain disulphide bond that spans approximately 60 amino acids. The polypeptide chain in each domain is folded into seven or eight antiparallel β strands that are arranged so that they form two opposing sheets. The disulphide bond and hydrophobic interactions link the two sheets. This compact structure is called the immunoglobulin fold (Fig. 3.8). Light chains contain one variable and one constant domain. Heavy chains contain one variable and three or four constant domains, depending on the class of antibody (Fig. 3.9).

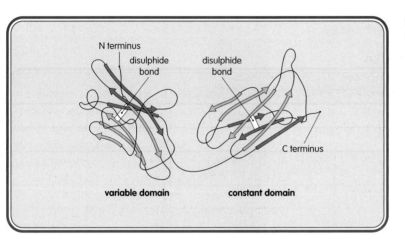

Fig. 3.8 Immunoglobulin fold structure of a light chain.

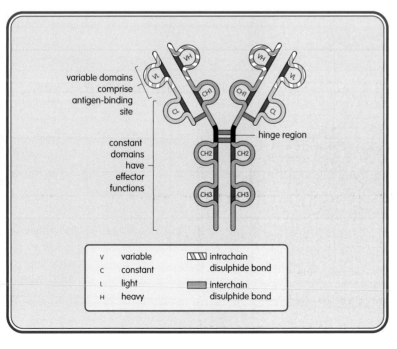

Fig. 3.9 Structure of an immunoglobulin, showing domains.

Structure of an Ig in relation to function

The variable domains (heavy and light chains)

Each variable domain has three hypervariable regions which are separated by framework regions. The hypervariable regions constitute the antigen-binding site of the Ig and therefore define the antigen specificity of a particular antibody. Because they are complementary to the structure of the epitope they bind, the hypervariable regions are also known as complementarity-determining regions (CDRs).

The hinge region and the constant domains

The heavy chains of IgG, IgA, and IgD have three constant domains and a hinge region. IgM and IgE heavy chains have four constant domains but lack a hinge region. The hinge region is a peptide sequence located between CH1 and CH2. It allows considerable movement of the Fab and Fc regions, thus allowing greater interaction with epitopes as well as maximal effector function. It is also the site of the disulphide bonds that hold the two heavy chains together. The number of interchain disulphide bonds varies depending on the Ig class/subclass. The most important constant domains functionally are the C-terminal domains, i.e. CH3 in IgG, IgA, and IgD; CH4 in IgM and IgE. Their functions reflect the functions of the different Ig classes (Fig. 3.10).

Properties of the five immunoglobulin classes					
	IgG	IgA	IgM	IgE	IgD
Physical properties					
molecular weight (D)	150 000	150 000 (monomer)	900 000 (pentamer)	190 000	150 000
serum concentration (mg/mL)	13.5*	3.5	1.5	0.0003	0.03
subunits	1	1/2	5	1	1
heavy chain	γ	α	μ	ε	δ
subclasses	4 (γ1, γ2, γ3, γ4)	2 (α1, α2)	—	—	—
Biological activities (are functions of the constant domains)					
present in secretions	×	✓	✓	×	×
crosses placenta	✓	×	×	×	×
complement fixation	✓ (classical pathway) (mainly IgG1 + IgG3)	✓ (alternative pathway)	✓ (classical pathway)	×	×
binding to phagocytic FcRs	✓ (mainly IgG1 + IgG3)	×	✓	×	×
binding to mast cell FcRs	×	×	×	✓	×
Other features					
main role	main circulatory Ig in secondary immune response	major Ig of secretions, e.g. saliva, breast milk, mucus	main Ig in primary immune response	role in allergy and antiparasitic response	expressed on virgin B cell membrane; function not known

*IgG subclasses are present in the following proportions: IgG1 IgG2 IgG3 IgG4
9 : 3 : 1 : 0.5
These figures also correspond to their serum concentrations in mg/mL.

Fig. 3.10 Properties of the five immunoglobulin classes.

Different immunoglobulins and their functions

Different Ig classes and subclasses are called *isotypes* and are specific to each species. Igs G, E, and D are monomeric. Secreted IgA (sIgA) is usually present as a dimer, and secreted IgM as a pentamer. The sIgA molecule is made up of two IgA monomers, a J chain, and a secretory piece. The IgA dimer (+ J chain) is produced by submucosal plasma cells and enters the mucosal epithelial cell via receptor-mediated endocytosis, binding to the poly-Ig receptor. Having passed from the basal to the luminal surface of the epithelial cell, the IgA dimer is secreted with part of the poly-Ig receptor (the secretory piece) still attached.

The functions of Igs are as follows:

- **Opsonization**—the antibody–antigen complex can bind to phagocytic cells via the Fc component of the antibody, facilitating phagocytosis.
- **Agglutination**—IgG and IgM are both capable of this, but IgM is more efficient, as it has a high valency (10 antigen-binding sites) and can therefore bind many epitopes at the same time, enhancing phagocytosis.
- **Neutralization**—by binding to the pathogen or its toxins, antibodies prevent their attachment to cells.
- **Antibody-dependent cell-mediated cytotoxicity** (ADCC)—the antibody–antigen complex can bind to cytotoxic cells (e.g. cytotoxic T cells, NK cells) via the Fc component of the antibody, thus targeting the antigen for destruction.
- **Complement activation**—IgG and IgM can activate the classical pathway; IgA can activate the alternative pathway.
- **Mast cell degranulation**—most of the body's IgE is bound to mast cells and basophils, and upon cross-linkage of the IgE, degranulation occurs.
- **Protection of the neonate**—transplacental passage of IgG and the secretion of sIgA in breast milk protect the newborn.

The following two definitions are important:

- **Allotype**—although we all have the same genes encoding our isotypes, there are multiple alleles for some loci, giving rise to different structural forms of certain isotypes, called allotypes. This term refers to differences within a species. For example, there are two variants of the IgA2 subclass.
- **Idiotype**—the variable domains of Igs, in addition to binding epitopes, can function as epitopes themselves: each epitope is referred to as an *idiotope*, and the sum of all the idiotopes of an antibody is called the idiotype.

The B cell surface antigen receptor

The B cell surface antigen receptor is membrane immunoglobulin (mIg) associated with two molecules of the Igα/Igβ heterodimer (Fig. 3.11).

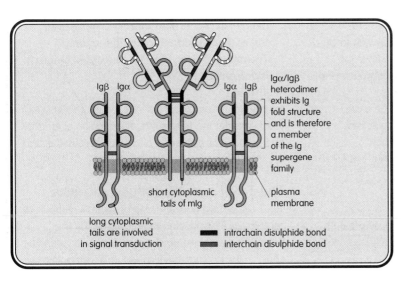

Fig. 3.11 Structure of the B cell surface antigen receptor. (mIg, membrane immunoglobulin.)

Igα/Igβ heterodimer exhibits Ig fold structure and is therefore a member of the Ig supergene family

short cytoplasmic tails of mIg

plasma membrane

long cytoplasmic tails are involved in signal transduction

▬ intrachain disulphide bond
▬ interchain disulphide bond

Igβ Igα — Igα Igβ

The extracellular portion of mIg is identical in structure to sIg. However, unlike sIg, mIg has transmembrane and cytoplasmic portions that anchor it to the membrane. Different Ig classes may be expressed on the same B cell and may indicate the stage of development of the B cell, e.g. a mature but antigenically unchallenged B cell expresses both mIgM and mIgD. However, the antigenic specificity of all of the mIg molecules is the same. Once antigen has bound mIg, the two Igα/Igβ heterodimers are responsible for signal transduction. They have longer cytoplasmic portions than mIg and can thus interact with intracellular enzymes.

- Describe the structure and functions of an immunoglobulin molecule.
- List the structural and functional differences between the five immunoglobulin classes.
- Define the terms isotype, allotype, idiotype, and idiotope.
- Summarize the concept of the immunoglobulin supergene family.

If asked to list the functions of immunoglobulins, categorize them either by *function*, as on p. 25, or by *class*, as in Fig. 3.10.

The immunoglobulin gene superfamily

The Ig domain structure is found in both the heavy and light chains, although these are separate peptides encoded by different genes. It has been found that molecules other than Igs show homology with the Ig domain structure. These molecules constitute the **immunoglobulin gene superfamily**. Examples include:

- Igα/Igβ heterodimer.
- T cell receptor.
- Major histocompatibility complex molecules.
- T cell accessory molecules such as CD4.
- Certain adhesion molecules, e.g. ICAM-1, ICAM-2, and VCAM-1.
- Poly-Ig receptor.

It is thought that the genes encoding these proteins were derived from a common ancestral gene encoding the Ig domain.

RECOGNITION MOLECULES: THE T CELL

Antigen recognition by T cells differs from antigen recognition by B cells:

- T cells recognize antigen only when it is associated with a molecule of the major histocompatibility complex (MHC).
- T cells recognize peptide fragments of an antigen in association with MHC molecules rather than its individual conformation. Therefore, antigen must be processed before it is presented to the T cell.

In order to understand T cell–antigen interaction, we must consider the T cell surface antigen receptor, MHC interactions, the pathways of antigen processing, and the role of accessory molecules.

The T cell surface antigen receptor

The T cell surface antigen receptor consists of the T cell receptor (TCR) associated with CD3. The TCR is a heterodimer, comprising α- and β-chains, or γ- and δ-chains. Each chain comprises two Ig-like domains: one variable and one constant. Also, three complementarity determining regions (CDRs, see p. 24) are present in each variable domain.

Approximately 95% of T cells express $\alpha\beta$ receptors. T cells expressing $\gamma\delta$ receptors are found particularly in epithelial tissues. CD3 is made up of five polypeptide chains that are arranged in the form of three dimers: $\gamma\varepsilon$, $\delta\varepsilon$, and $\zeta\zeta$ (found in 90% of CD3 molecules) or $\zeta\eta$. The γ-, δ-, and ε-chains, but not the ζ- and η-chains, are members of the Ig gene superfamily. The TCR recognizes and binds antigen, and CD3, functionally analogous to the Igα/Igβ heterodimer in B cells, is involved in signal transduction (Fig. 3.12).

The major histocompatibility complex (MHC)

The MHC is a cluster of tightly linked genes. In humans, the MHC is also called the HLA (human leucocyte antigen) complex and is located on chromosome 6.

The genes of the MHC

The genes are divided into three regions, each region encoding one of the three classes of the MHC: class I, class II, and class III (Fig. 3.13).

The genes of the MHC have two important features:
- They exhibit a high degree of *polymorphism*, i.e. there are a large number of alleles at most loci. Consequently, MHC molecules exhibit considerable diversity, e.g. there are more than 50 distinct alleles for HLA-B.
- The loci are tightly linked (we inherit sets of alleles, each called a *haplotype*, one from our father and one from our mother). The alleles exhibit codominance: both the maternal and paternal alleles are expressed. Individuals are generally heterozygous at most loci.

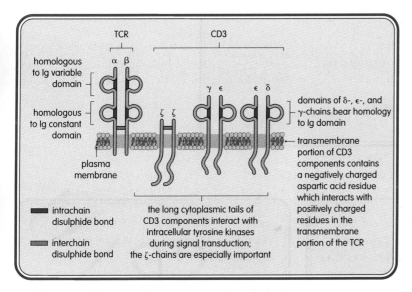

Fig. 3.12 Structure of the T cell surface antigen receptor.

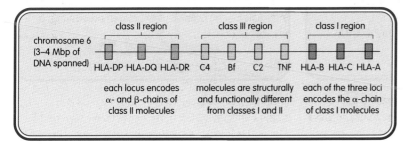

Fig. 3.13 Genetic organization of the human leucocyte antigen (HLA) complex. Only the classical genes are shown for class I and class II.

Structure and function of the MHC

Class I and class II MHC molecules are glycoproteins expressed on the cell surface and consist of cytoplasmic, transmembrane, and extracellular portions (Figs 3.14–3.16).

Both class I and class II molecules exhibit broad specificity in their binding of peptide. Peptides isolated from the clefts of class I molecules are 8–9 amino acids in length, whereas those from class II molecules are 13–18 amino acids in length. Class II molecules can bind longer peptides because their peptide-binding cleft is more open. The polymorphism of the MHC is largely concentrated in the peptide-binding cleft.

Class I molecules are normally found on all nucleated cells, and present endogenous antigen to CD8+ T cells. Class II molecules are found on antigen-presenting cells (APCs), and present exogenous antigen to CD4+ T cells. Class III molecules include complement components (C4, C2, factor B) and tumour necrosis factor.

Antigen processing and presentation

MHC molecules bind peptides. The antigen must therefore be processed before it can be presented in conjunction with the MHC molecule.

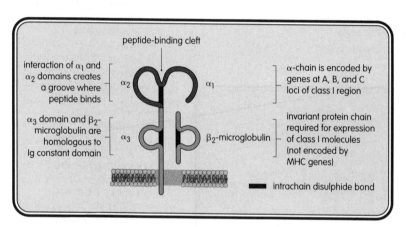

peptide-binding cleft

interaction of α_1 and α_2 domains creates a groove where peptide binds

α_2 α_1

α-chain is encoded by genes at A, B, and C loci of class I region

α_3 domain and β_2-microglobulin are homologous to Ig constant domain

α_3 β_2-microglobulin

invariant protein chain required for expression of class I molecules (not encoded by MHC genes)

intrachain disulphide bond

Fig. 3.14 Structure of a major histocompatibility complex (MHC) class I molecule.

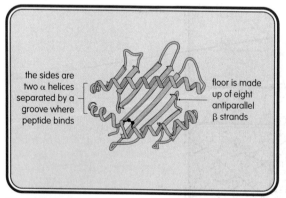

the sides are two α helices separated by a groove where peptide binds

floor is made up of eight antiparallel β strands

Fig. 3.15 Peptide-binding cleft of a major histocompatibility complex (MHC) class I molecule as seen from above.

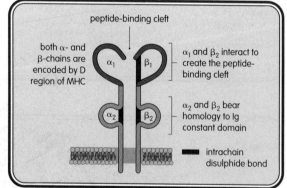

peptide-binding cleft

both α- and β-chains are encoded by D region of MHC

α_1 β_1

α_1 and β_2 interact to create the peptide-binding cleft

α_2 β_2

α_2 and β_2 bear homology to Ig constant domain

intrachain disulphide bond

Fig. 3.16 Structure of a major histocompatibility complex (MHC) class II molecule.

Antigen processing

There are two different pathways of antigen processing (Fig. 3.17).

Antigen presentation

In general, two types of cell present antigen to T cells:

- APCs—by convention, APCs are defined as cells that can process and present antigen to CD4+ T cells in association with class II molecules. They include Langerhans' cells, interdigitating cells, dendritic cells, macrophages, and B cells. These cells express high levels of class II MHC molecules.
- Cells presenting antigen in association with class I molecules to CD8+ T cells—these include virus-infected cells and 'altered self cells', e.g. cancer cells.

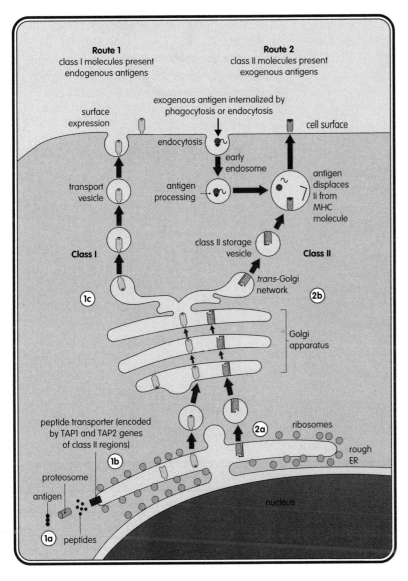

Fig. 3.17 The two routes of antigen processing. **Route 1:** (1a) antigen is degraded within the proteosome, a complex of proteolytic enzymes, two subunits of which are encoded by the class II region (LMP2 and LMP7); (1b) the resulting peptides are transported into the rough endoplasmic reticulum (rough ER), where they associate with newly synthesized class I molecules; (1c) the class I molecule with peptide bound is transported via the Golgi complex to the cell surface and expressed. **Route 2:** (2a) the invariant chain (Ii) occupies the peptide-binding cleft of class II molecules in rough ER, preventing binding of endogenous proteins; (2b) the class II molecule is transported via the Golgi appartus to an endosomal/lysosomal compartment, where low pH causes dissociation of Ii, allowing binding of peptides derived from exogenous antigen.

MHC restriction

T cells only recognize antigen in association with self-MHC (self-MHC restriction). CD8⁺ T cells only recognize antigen if it is presented in association with class I MHC molecules. CD4⁺ T cells only recognize antigen if it is presented in association with class II MHC molecules. Therefore, CD8⁺ T cells are said to be class I MHC restricted and CD4⁺ T cells, class II MHC restricted.

Accessory molecules

As well as the TCR, CD3, and MHC molecules, other 'accessory' molecules such as CD4 and CD8 play an important role in the T cell–antigen interaction. CD4 and CD8 have two important functions:

- They bind MHC class II and class I molecules, respectively, thereby strengthening the T cell–antigen interaction.
- They function as signal transducers.

GENERATION OF ANTIGEN RECEPTOR DIVERSITY

The B cell

More than 10^8 antibody specificities can be generated. The random generation of diversity has a genetic basis. The κ and λ light chains and the heavy chain are encoded by a number of *gene segments* (Figs 3.18 and 3.19).

The V, D (heavy chain only), and J exons together encode the variable regions of the Ig molecule, and the C exons encode the constant regions. Heavy chain C gene segments are clusters of exons, each of which encodes either a domain or hinge region of the constant region.

During B cell maturation, rearrangement ensures that the clonal progeny of each B cell produce Ig of a single specificity. Rearrangement is complete and functional Ig chains are produced before the B cell encounters antigen (Figs 3.20 and 3.21).

- Describe the differences in antigen recognition by B cells and T cells.
- Summarize the genetics of the MHC and its role in antigen presentation to T cells.
- What are the two different pathways of antigen processing?
- Describe the concept of MHC restriction.

Gene segments encoding immunoglobulin chains in humans						
Ig chain	Location	Encoded by	No. of gene segments			
			V	D	J	C
κ light chain	chromosome 2	V, J, and C segments	~100	—	5	1
λ light chain	chromosome 22	V, J, and C segments	~100	—	6	6
heavy chain	chromosome 14	V, D, J, and C segments	75–250	30	6	9

Fig. 3.18 The gene segments encoding immunoglobulin chains in humans.

Allelic exclusion

This is the process whereby a B cell expresses only one set of heavy chain genes and only one set of light chain genes thus ensuring that the antigenic specificity of the two halves of the Ig molecule is the same. Production of a functional heavy or light chain prevents rearrangement of the other sets of genes.

Class switching

This is the process whereby a single B cell can produce different classes of Ig that have the same specificity. The mechanism is not well understood but involves 'switch sites'—DNA sequences located upstream from each heavy chain C gene segment (except C_δ). Possible mechanisms include:

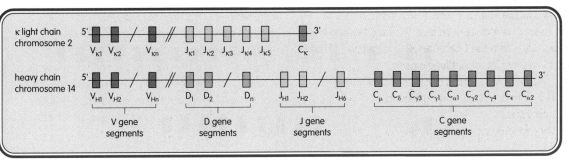

Fig. 3.19 Germline organization of the human κ (kappa) light and heavy chain gene segments.

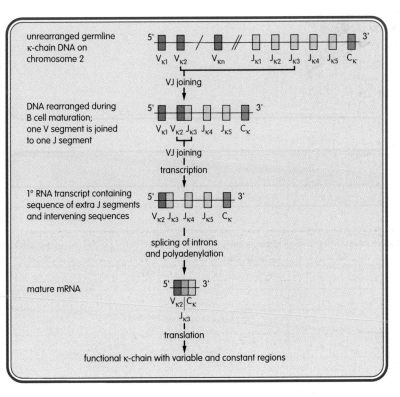

Fig. 3.20 κ light chain gene rearrangements.

- Differential splicing of the primary transcript (as in Fig. 3.21).
- A looping out and deletion of intervening heavy chain C gene segments (and introns).
- Exchange of C gene segments between chromosomes.

This process underlies the class switch from IgM in the primary response, to IgG in the secondary response (see Fig. 3.1). Cytokines are important in controlling the switch.

Generation of diversity

The presence of multiple V, D (heavy chain only),

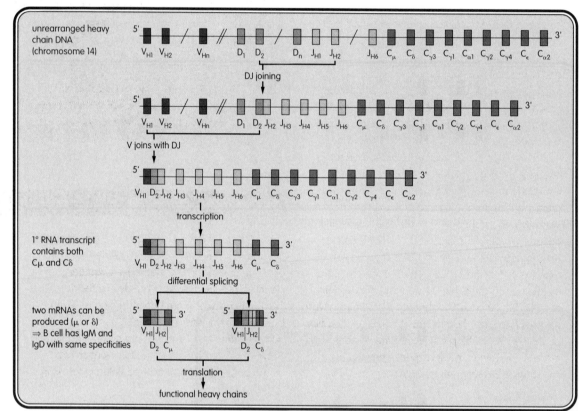

Fig. 3.21 Heavy chain gene rearrangements.

Calculation of antibody diversity			
Mechanism of diversity	**Number of combinations**		
	κ **light chain**	λ **light chain**	**heavy chain**
random joining of V, D, and J segments (V × J for light chains, V × J × D for the heavy chain)	100 × 5 = 500	100 × 6 = 600	75 × 30 × 6 = 13 500
any light chain can associate with any heavy chain	$(500 + 600) \times 13\,500 = 1.5 \times 10^7$		
junctional flexibility	✓	✓	✓
N-nucleotide addition	✗	✗	✓
somatic hypermutation	✓	✓	✓
The extent of the contribution of the last three mechanisms to antibody diversity is not known but is considered significant			

Fig. 3.22 Calculation of antibody diversity.

and J gene segments and the apparently random selection of these segments generates considerable diversity. Other mechanisms generating diversity include:

- **Junctional flexibility**—the slight variations in the position of segmental joining.
- **N-nucleotide addition**—the addition of nucleotides to the D-J and the V-DJ joints. Up to 15 nucleotides can be added in a reaction catalysed by terminal deoxynucleotidyl transferase. This process only occurs in heavy chains. Both junctional flexibility and N-nucleotide addition can disrupt the reading frame, leading to non-functional rearrangements. However, as some rearrangements are productive, they potentially increase antibody diversity. The V-J, V-DJ, and VD-J joints all fall within CDR3 of the Ig heavy and light chain variable regions. Therefore, diversity generated at these joints by junctional flexibility and N-nucleotide addition has a great impact on the antigen specificity of the Ig molecule.
- **Somatic hypermutation**—occurs after contact with antigen. During the course of a primary immune response, point mutations occur in the variable region exons of the Ig molecule. The resultant Ig molecules may have higher or lower affinities for antigen, but those with higher affinities are positively selected because of clonal antigen drive. Antibodies produced later in the primary immune response and in the secondary immune response have an increased affinity for antigen (*affinity maturation*).

Antibody diversity can be calculated (Fig. 3.22).

The T cell

Random combination of V, D, and J segments occurs (α- and γ-chain variable domains are encoded by V and J segments; β- and δ-chain variable domains are encoded by V, D, and J segments). N-nucleotide addition and junctional flexibility occur. Somatic hypermutation does not occur, reducing the chances of self-reactive T cells arising and thus maintaining tolerance to self.

- What are the mechanisms whereby antigen receptor diversity is generated?
- Summarize the principles of allelic exclusion, class switching, and affinity maturation.

HUMORAL IMMUNITY

The initiators of the humoral immune response are antibodies. They are particularly efficient at eliminating extracellular pathogens. Antigen can be cleared from the host by a variety of effector mechanisms, which are dependent on antibody class or isotype (see also p. 25):

- Activation of the complement system, leading to lysis or opsonization of the microorganism.
- Antibody-dependent cell-mediated cytotoxicity (ADCC).
- Neutralization of bacterial toxins and viruses.
- Mucosal immunity (IgA-mediated).

An effective humoral immune response usually involves B cells, activated T helper (Th) cells, and APCs (Fig. 3.23).

Some antigens—e.g. lipopolysaccharides from Gram-negative bacterial cell walls—stimulate B cells directly and do not require T cell help. These are known as T cell-independent antigens.

Generation of antigen receptor diversity is likely to be examined in the essay section of the exam. Be able to explain the genetic basis of receptor diversity and list the additional mechanisms. Remember to mention the T cell receptor!

- Describe the processes leading to the development of an effective humoral immune response.

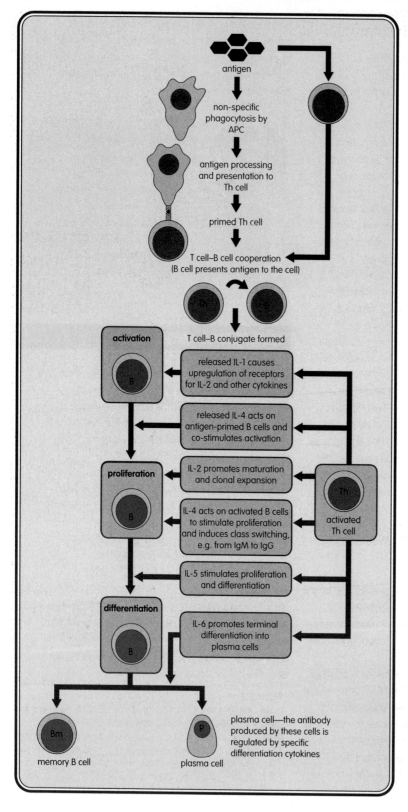

Fig. 3.23 Overview of the humoral immune response. Most antigens require T cell help to induce an immune response (T-cell dependent antigens). Antigen is phagocytosed non-specifically by antigen-presenting cells (APCs), which process and present the antigen to CD4+ T cells in conjunction with MHC class II molecules. Antigen also interacts with B cell membrane IgD or IgM receptors. Primed T helper (Th) cells then interact with B cells, which present antigen to them. This induces expression of CD40L on the Th cell membrane, which binds to CD40 on the B cell membrane and is the single most potent activating signal to B cells, which divide and differentiate. Various cytokines released by Th cells stimulate the different stages of this process.

CELL-MEDIATED IMMUNITY

Cell-mediated immunity is mediated by T lymphocytes, macrophages, and neutrophils. The cell-mediated immune system is involved in the elimination of:

- Intracellular pathogens.
- Tumour cells.
- Virus-infected cells.
- Foreign grafts.

T cells

T cell development and maturation takes place in the thymus (Fig. 3.24). The T cell population can be classified on the basis of either function or expression of cell surface molecules.

Positive and negative selection of T cells

Positive and negative selection of T cells occurs in the thymus.

Positive selection of T cells

Positive selection occurs in the cortex and results in selection of T cells that are capable of binding self-MHC molecules and confers MHC restriction upon T cells, ensuring that the selected T cells only recognize antigen in conjunction with either class I or class II MHC molecules. The developing CD4+ CD8+ T cells interact with thymic epithelial cells, which express high levels of class I and class II MHC molecules.

T cells that do not interact with the MHC molecules are presumed to undergo apoptosis, as they do not receive a protective signal as a result of the TCR–MHC interaction.

Negative selection of T cells

Some of the T cells that survive positive selection have high affinity for MHC molecules. These CD4+ CD8+ T cells undergo negative selection. Negative selection is thought to be mediated by dendritic cells and macrophages, which express high levels of class I and class II MHC molecules. 'Self-reactive' T cells expressing high-affinity receptors for self-MHC alone, or for self-MHC and antigen, interact with the MHC molecules on dendritic cells and macrophages and apoptose. Negative selection occurs in the corticomedullary junction and medulla of the thymus.

Positive and negative selection results in T cells that moderately recognize foreign antigens in conjunction with self-MHC molecules.

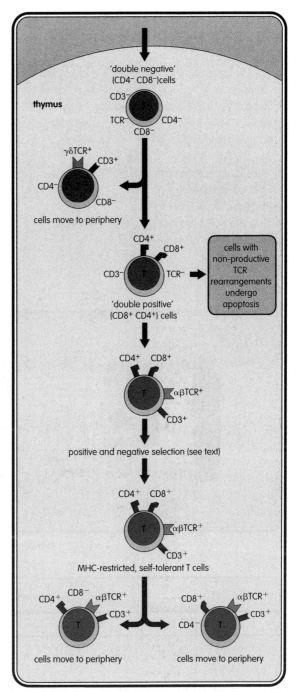

Fig. 3.24 Pathway for T cell development in the thymus. On entering the thymus, T cells are Thy1+. Most of the T cells in the thymus die due to non-productive T cell receptor arrangements (when they undergo apoptosis) or because they fail positive or negative selection. T cells that move out of the thymus into the periphery are of three distinct types: CD4+ αβ cells, CD8+ αβ cells, and CD4− CD8− γδ cells. The first two cell types constitute most of the peripheral T cells.

35

T helper cells

Th cells play a key role in the development of the immune response:

- They are required for normal B cell function (see pp. 34–35).
- They determine the epitopes that are targeted by the immune system via their interactions with antigen in conjunction with class II MHC molecules on APCs (Fig. 3.25).
- They determine the nature of the immune response directed against target antigens, e.g. cytotoxic T cell response or antibody response.
- They promote proliferation of the appropriate cell type.

Most Th cells are CD4+, but can be CD8+. Th cells can be divided into three subsets on the basis of the cytokines they secrete:

- Th0.
- Th1.
- Th2.

Th0 cells arise as a result of initial short-term stimulation of naive T cells. They are capable of secreting a broad spectrum of cytokines. Prolonged stimulation results in the emergence of Th1 and Th2 subsets. The cytokines released by the Th1 and Th2 subsets modulate one another's secretion. The different cytokine profiles of the Th1 and Th2 subsets reflect their different immunological functions (Fig. 3.26).

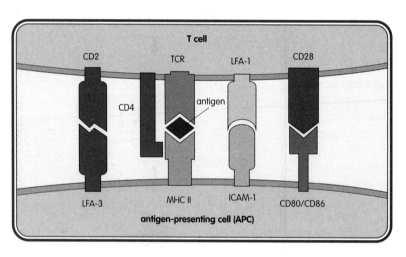

Fig. 3.25 Molecules involved in the interaction between T cells and antigen-presenting cells (APCs). (TCR, T cell receptor; LFA-1/LFA-3, leucocyte function antigen 1/3; ICAM-1, intercellular adhesion molecule 1.)

Differences between Th1 and Th2 cells		
	Th1 cells	**Th2 cells**
cytokines secreted	IL-2, IL-3, IFN-γ, TNF-β	IL-3, IL-4, IL-5, IL-10, IL-13
functions	• responsible for classical cell-mediated immunity reactions such as delayed-type hypersensitivity and cytotoxic T cell activation • involved in responses to intracellular pathogens • activate macrophages	• promote B cell activation • involved in allergic diseases and responses to helminthic infections • induce rise in IgE and eosinophil levels

Fig. 3.26 Differences between T helper (Th) cell subsets—Th1 and Th2.

Cytotoxic T cells

Most cytotoxic T (Tc) lymphocytes are CD8+ and recognize antigen in conjunction with class I MHC molecules. They lyse target cells via a variety of mechanisms (Fig. 3.27).

Suppressor T cells

Although both CD4+ and CD8+ T cells are capable of suppressing or terminating immune responses, they probably do not exist as functionally distinct entities.

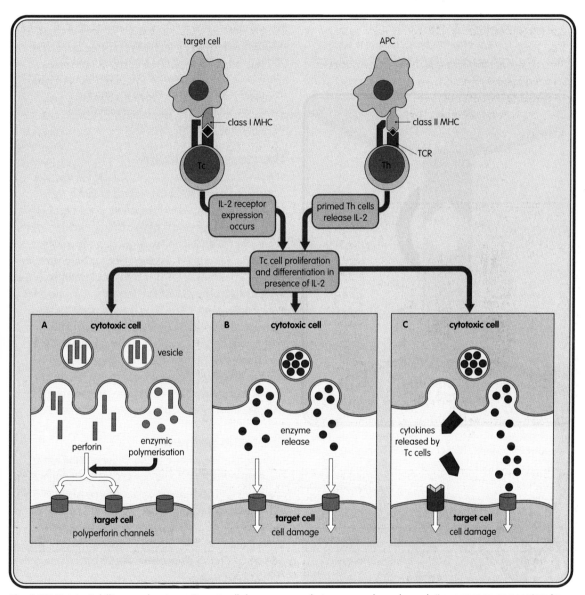

Fig. 3.27 Cytotoxic killing mechanisms. Target cell damage occurs in three main ways. (A) Calcium influx leads to a discharge of granule contents; monomers of perforin, a protein present in the granules, insert into the target cell membrane and polymerize to form a transmembrane channel. This induces fragmentation of the cell. (B) Lytic substances, such as degradative enzymes, may enter via these channels and cause damage to the target cell. (C) Cytokines, such as TNFβ and IFN-γ released by Tc cells, seem to induce apoptosis of the target cell. The exact mechanism is unknown. (Tc, cytotoxic T cell; APC, antigen-presenting cell; Th, T helper.)

Superantigens

Superantigens, such as certain staphylococcal toxins, are capable of activating T cells non-specifically by binding simultaneously to the class II MHC molecule and the Vβ domain of the TCR (Fig. 3.28). Because superantigens bind outside the antigen-binding cleft of the TCR, they can activate any T cell expressing a particular Vβ sequence. As the number of Vβ sequences is limited, any one superantigen is capable of activating approximately 5% of the T cell population.

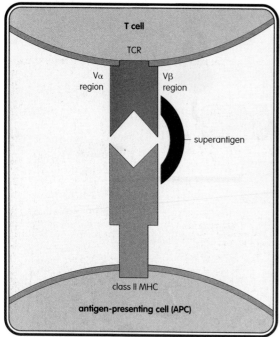

Fig. 3.28 Superantigen binding to the T cell receptor (TCR) and major histocompatibility complex (MHC) class II molecules. The superantigen binds non-specifically to the TCR (via the Vβ region) and class II MHC molecules.

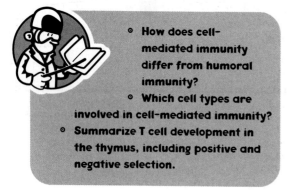

- **How does cell-mediated immunity differ from humoral immunity?**
- **Which cell types are involved in cell-mediated immunity?**
- **Summarize T cell development in the thymus, including positive and negative selection.**

THE COMPLEMENT SYSTEM

The complement system is a group of over 20 serum glycoproteins, synthesized principally by hepatocytes. Many of the complement components circulate in the serum as proenzymes (functionally inactive enzymes) and require proteolytic cleavage for activation. Once a component is activated, it catalyses the next step of the pathway. Components only remain in the activated state for a short time. There are three pathways of complement activation—the classical, the lectin, and the alternative pathways—which terminate in a common final pathway (Fig. 3.29).

The classical pathway

Antigen-bound IgG and IgM can activate the classical pathway via their CH2 or CH3 domains. IgM is more efficient than IgG. The first component of the classical pathway, C1, exists as a complex, $C1qr_2s_2$, which consists of one C1q molecule and two molecules each of the monomers C1s and C1r. Binding to the Ig domain occurs via the C1q component. This results in autocatalysis of the two C1r molecules, which then cleave the C1s molecules to their active form. C1s acts on both C4 and C2. C4b, a cleavage product of C4, binds to the surface of the antigen and acts as a binding site for C2. Bound C2 is then cleaved by C1s, and the larger fragment, C2a, remains bound to C4b to form a complex, C4b2a (C3 convertase). C4b2a cleaves C3. The C3b generated binds C4b2a to form the C4b2a3b complex (C5 convertase).

The lectin pathway

Mannan-binding protein (MBP) is found in the serum and bears structural homology to C1q. It is thought to associate with MBP-associated serine protease (MASP), which bears some homology to C1r and C1s. MBP binds to carbohydrate groups on the surface of bacteria. Upon binding of MBP, MASP is activated. MASP then acts on C4 and C2 to generate the C3 convertase of the classical pathway.

The alternative pathway

C3 contains a labile thioester bond that is susceptible to spontaneous hydrolysis. The C3b generated is deposited on host and microbial surfaces. Certain features of microbial surfaces allow persistence of C3b:

- They lack regulatory molecules that inactivate C3b (these are present in eukaryotic cell membranes).
- On microbial surfaces, C3b tends to bind factor B rather than factor H (an inhibitory molecule).

The binding of factor B to C3b allows factor B to act as a substrate for factor D. Cleavage of factor B results in the formation of the C3bBb complex (C3 convertase), which is stabilized by the protein properdin. As in the classical pathway, C3 convertase cleaves C3, and the C3b generated binds C3bBb to form C3bBb3b (C5 convertase).

The common terminal pathway

The non-enzymatic C3b component of the C5 convertase binds C5 and alters its conformation so that the enzymatically active portion (C4b2a or C3bBb) can cleave it. C5b sequentially binds C6, C7, C8, and C9. C5b67 inserts into the cell membrane, and C8 binds to this membrane-bound complex. C9 is a perforin-like molecule and its binding to C5b678 and subsequent polymerization creates an ion-permeable pore, resulting in osmotic lysis of the cell. This final stage of the complement pathway, the C5b6789 complex, is also called the membrane-attack complex (MAC).

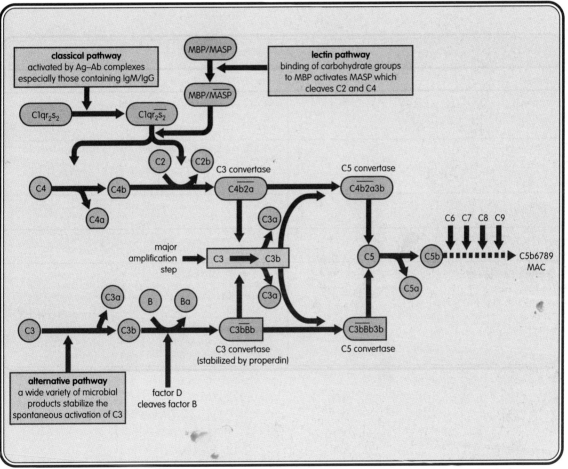

Fig. 3.29 The classical, lectin, and alternative pathways of complement activation. Proteolytic cleavage of the complement components results in fragments that are designated 'a' (smaller fragments) or 'b' (larger fragments). The exception to this is C2, where the larger fragment is designated 'a' and the smaller fragment 'b'. The larger fragment binds to the surface of the antigen, and the smaller one diffuses away. An enzymatically active component has a bar drawn above its notation, e.g. the enzymatically active component of C4a2a3b is C4a2a.

The transmembrane pores created by C5b67 and C5b678, although not as large as those created by the MAC, can result in lysis of anucleate cells such as red blood cells, which are less resistant to lysis. In addition, C5b67 can insert into the membranes of neighbouring, healthy cells, causing 'reactive lysis'.

Amplification

In both the classical and alternative pathways, C3 convertase can generate many hundreds of C3b molecules. This is the major amplification step of the complement pathway.

Functions of complement

The products of the complement pathway play an important role in both adaptive and innate immunity (Fig. 3.30).

Inhibitors of complement

Inhibitors of the complement pathway are important in regulating its activity and preventing complement-mediated damage of healthy cells (Fig. 3.31).

Functions of complement	
Function	**Notes**
cell lysis	MAC makes pores in cell membranes; effective against Gram-negative bacteria; nucleated cells more resistant to lysis as they can apparently endocytose MAC
inflammation	C3a, C4a, and C5a are anaphylatoxins and cause degranulation of mast cells and basophils; C3a and C5a are chemotactic for neutrophils and monocytes; C5a is much more potent than C3a and is also is a highly efficient phagocyte activator
opsonization	C3b acts as an opsonin and enhances phagocytosis of antigen by cells expressing complement receptors
viral neutralization	various mechanisms—e.g. MAC induces lysis of enveloped viruses, C3b coats viral particles and prevents their attachment to target cells
solubilization and clearance of immune complexes	solubilization—classical pathway prevents immune complex precipitation; alternative pathway facilitates solubilization of those already precipitated; C3 is incorporated into immune complex lattices and disrupts them, reducing their size
	clearance—immune complexes are coated with C3b, which binds to CR1 on red blood cells; on passage through spleen, immune complexes are removed and phagocytosed

Fig. 3.30 Functions of complement.

Inhibitors of the complement pathway	
Inhibitor	**Action**
C1 inhibitor	binds C1r$_2$s$_2$, causing it to dissociate from C1q
membrane cofactor protein (MCP)* complement receptor type 1(CR1)* C4b-binding protein (C4bBP)* factor H*	prevent assembly of C3 convertase by: (A) binding C4b and preventing association with C2a (classical pathway); (B) binding C3b and preventing association with factor B (alternative pathway) MCP and CR1 act on both pathways, C4bBP acts only on the classical pathway, and factor H acts only on the alternative pathway
factor I	cleaves C4b (classical pathway) and C3b (alternative pathway) once they have been bound by MCP, CR1, C4bBP, or factor H
decay-accelerator factor (DAF)*	accelerates decay of C3 convertase in both pathways
S protein	binds C5b67 and prevents insertion into cell membrane; important in preventing reactive lysis
homologous restriction factor	prevents formation and insertion of MAC into membranes of autologous cells

Fig. 3.31 Inhibitors of the complement pathway. *These are members of the regulators of complement activation (RCA) family and are all encoded by a tightly linked cluster of genes on chromosome 1. The RCA family of proteins is characterized by the presence of repeating sequences 60 amino acids long, called short consensus repeats.

- **Summarize the different pathways of complement activation.**
- **List the functions of complement.**
- **How is complement activity regulated?**

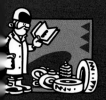

4. The Immune System in Disease

RESPONSE TO TISSUE DAMAGE

Inflammation is a non-specific response evoked by tissue injury. The aims of the inflammatory process are:
- Removal of the causative agent, e.g. microbes or toxins.
- Removal of dead tissue.
- Replacement of dead tissue with normal tissue, or scar formation.

Acute inflammation
Acute inflammation is the immediate response to cell injury. It is of short duration (a few hours to a few days).

Vascular changes
Tissue injury results in the release of chemical mediators that act on local blood vessels. The main changes which occur are:
- Vasodilatation—this results in increased blood flow and hence redness and heat.
- Slowing of the circulation and increased vascular permeability—this results in the formation of an inflammatory exudate (extravascular fluid with a high protein content) and hence swelling.
- Entry of inflammatory cells, especially neutrophils.

Leucocyte extravasation
Neutrophils adhere to the vessel wall and then pass between the endothelial cells into the tissues. This is a multistep process involving:
- Margination.
- Diapedesis (extravasation).
- Chemotaxis

Margination
Margination is the adherence of the neutrophils to the vessel wall. It is mediated by cell adhesion molecules (CAMs) on inflammatory and endothelial cells (Fig. 4.1). CAMs may be members of the immunoglobulin gene superfamily, the selectin family, or the integrin family. A variety of inflammatory mediators modify the expression or alter the affinity of CAMs.

Cell adhesion molecules (CAMs) involved in margination of neutrophils				
Margination phase	Neutrophil cell adhesion molecule	Distribution	Endothelium cell adhesion molecule	Distribution
phase 1	L-selectin binds specific carbohydrate groups on endothelium	constitutively expressed; increased affinity after exposure to chemotactic factors	P-selectin and E-selectin both bind sialyl Lewis X antigen	P-selectin—inducible; stored in Wiebel-Palade bodies within endothelial cells; comes up in minutes E-selectin—inducible; has to be newly synthesized; comes up in hours
phase 2	MAC-1 and LFA-1—β_2 integrins—bind ICAM-1	inducible; stored in cytoplasmic vesicles (neutrophils cannot synthesize new proteins); therefore come up quickly	ICAM-1, a member of the Ig superfamily, binds LFA-1 and MAC-1	constitutively expressed; increased expression due to action of cytokines, e.g. IL-1 and TNF-α

Fig. 4.1 Cell adhesion molecules (CAMs) involved in margination of neutrophils. (MAC, membrane attack complex; LFA-1, leucocyte function antigen 1; ICAM-1, intercell adhesion molecule 1; IL-1, interleukin 1; TNF-α, tumour vecrosis factor-α.)

Two phases of margination are recognized:
- Phase I is characterized by weak, selectin-mediated binding, and results in the 'rolling' of neutrophils along the vessel wall.
- During phase II, neutrophils express integrins, which bind to molecules on the endothelium, resulting in a much stronger interaction.

Diapedesis

The tight, integrin-mediated binding of the neutrophil to the endothelium facilitates its emigration between the endothelial cells and into the tissue.

Chemotaxis

Neutrophils are attracted to the site of tissue damage by the release of chemotactic agents. These include:
- Complement products, especially C5a and C3a.
- Cytokines, especially IL-8.
- Platelet-activating factor (PAF).
- Arachidonic acid breakdown products, especially leukotriene B_4 (LTB_4).
- Fibrin and collagen fragments.
- N-formylmethionine residues (exclusively of bacterial origin).

In order to successfully interact with the extracellular matrix, neutrophils must express β_1 integrins, a set of adhesion molecules that can bind to collagen, laminin, etc. Phagocytosis of foreign particles and release of enzymes then occurs (see Chapter 3). Leucocytes may release potentially harmful proteases and metabolites during chemotaxis and phagocytosis.

Chemical mediators of inflammation

A variety of chemical mediators are produced. They usually have short half-lives and are rapidly inactivated by a variety of systems.

Stored mediators

Histamine released from mast cells, basophils, and platelets is responsible for the increased vascular permeability and also causes vasodilatation.

Synthesized mediators

Prostaglandins (PGs) and leukotrienes (LTs) are derived from the metabolism of arachadonic acid. PAF is also an important mediator (Fig. 4.2).

Cytokines

Cytokines such as IL-8, IL-1, and tumour necrosis factor-α (TNF-α) are also released. They act to:
- Induce PGI_2 production.
- Induce expression of CAMs on the endothelium, thus enhancing leucocyte adhesion.
- Induce PAF synthesis.
- Attract neutrophils to the area of injury.
- Mediate the development of the acute phase response.
- Stimulate fibroblast proliferation and increase collagen synthesis.

The complement system

This is discussed in Chapter 3.

The kinin system

The kinin system is activated by contact with Hageman factor (factor XII), ultimately resulting in the release of bradykinin (Fig. 4.3). Bradykinin causes an increase in vascular permeability and mediates pain.

The coagulation system

The coagulation system can also be activated by Hageman factor (factor XII) (see Chapter 23) resulting in the formation of insoluble fibrin from fibrinogen. In this process, fibrinopeptides are produced. These increase vascular permeability and are chemotactic for neutrophils. Thrombin (which converts fibrinogen into fibrin) also promotes fibroblast proliferation and leucocyte adhesion.

The fibrinolytic system

Tissue plasminogen activator (t-PA) is released from endothelial cells and leucocytes, and converts plasminogen into plasmin. Hageman factor, kallikrein, and high-molecular-weight kininogen (HMWK) are also capable of this. Plasmin has several functions in the inflammatory process, including activation of complement via C3 and cleavage of fibrin to form 'fibrin degradation products', which may increase vascular permeability. A summary of the mediators of acute inflammation is shown in Fig. 4.4.

Results of acute inflammation

The results of acute inflammation are shown in Fig. 4.5.

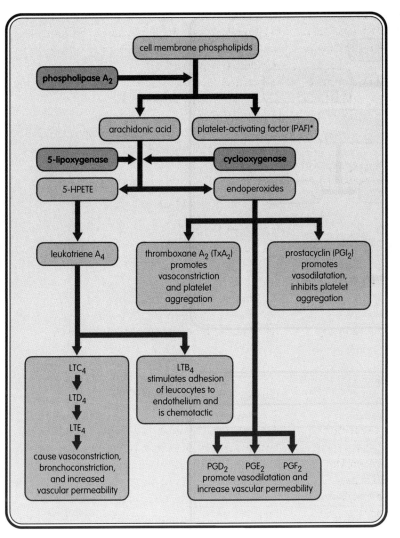

Fig. 4.2 Formation and action of some of the mediators involved in inflammation. *PAF (platelet-activating factor) is also produced by mast cells and basophils. It causes vasodilatation, increased vascular permeability, and platelet aggregation. It is 1000 times more potent than histamine.

Chronic inflammation

Chronic inflammation arises:

- When the causative agent cannot be eliminated and antigenic persistence occurs.
- As a result of persistent autoimmune reactions, e.g. systemic lupus erythematosus (SLE) and rheumatoid arthritis.
- Due to immune responses directed against certain microorganisms, e.g. *Mycobacterium tuberculosis*.

The main features are:

- Ongoing inflammation.
- Tissue destruction.
- Healing.

The key cells of chronic inflammation are:

- Macrophages.
- Lymphocytes.
- Plasma cells.

This is in marked contrast to acute inflammation, which is characterized by neutrophilic inflammation and vascular changes such as increased permeability and vasodilatation. An overview of chronic inflammation is shown in Fig. 4.6.

In chronic inflammation, macrophage numbers are increased by:

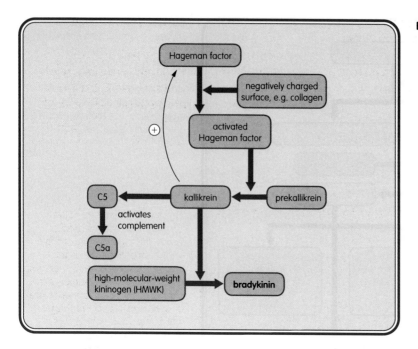

Fig. 4.3 Formation of bradykinin.

Mediators of acute inflammation	
Action	**Mediators**
increased vascular permeability	histamine, bradykinin, C3a, C5a, leukotrienes C_4, D_4, E_4, PAF
vasodilatation	histamine, prostaglandins, PAF
pain	bradykinin, prostaglandins
leucocyte adhesion	LTB_4, IL-1, TNF-α, C5a
leucocyte chemotaxis	IL-8, LTB_4, C5a
acute phase response	IL-1, TNF-α, IL-6
tissue damage	proteases and free radicals released by neutrophils

Fig. 4.4 Mediators of acute inflammation.

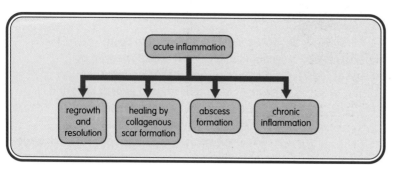

Fig. 4.5 Results of acute inflammation.

- Monocyte recruitment via chemotactic factors, e.g. C5a and platelet-derived growth factor (PDGF).
- Local division of macrophages.
- Migration inhibition factor (MIF), which prevents macrophage migration away from the site of inflammation.

Macrophage secretory products mediate characteristic features of chronic inflammation:

- Tissue damage via proteases and oxygen radicals
- Revascularization via angiogenic factors.
- Fibroblast migration and proliferation via growth factors (e.g. PGDF) and cytokines (IL-2, TNF-α).
- Collagen synthesis via growth factors (e.g. PGDF) and cytokines (IL-1, TNF-α).
- Remodelling via collagenases.

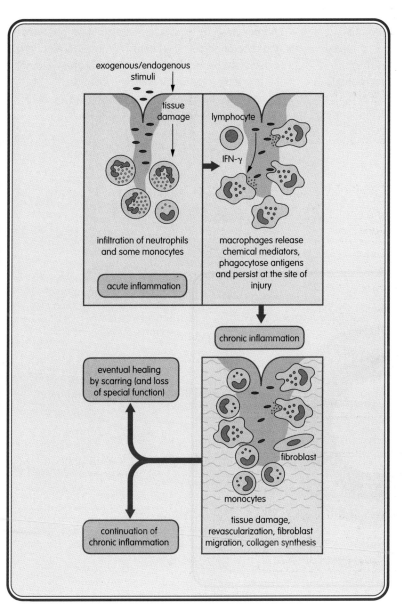

Fig. 4.6 Development of the chronic inflammatory process. Tissue damage stimulates rapid infiltration of neutrophils and vascular changes. Some monocytes may be present at the injury site after 48–72 hours. Monocytes are transformed into macrophages, which may be activated by, for example, IFN-γ released from sensitized T cells, or bacterial endotoxins. These 'activated' macrophages have greater phagocytic and killing ability, and can secrete a wide variety of chemical mediators. If inflammation is short-lived, the macrophages die or leave the area of injury. If inflammation persists, macrophages and lymphocytes remain at the injury site, resulting in chronic inflammation. Macrophage numbers increase, and the products they secrete produce characteristic features of chronic inflammation.

47

Lymphocytes and plasma cells are also present at the site of inflammation. Plasma cells secrete antibodies against either foreign antigen or altered host cell components.

Inflammation in disease

The inflammatory response is essentially a protective one. Under certain circumstances, however, it may prove to be destructive to the host. Antigenic persistence results in the continued activation and accumulation of macrophages. This leads to the formation of epithelioid cells (slightly modified macrophages) and granuloma formation (Fig. 4.7). Multinucleate giant cells, which arise from the fusion of several macrophages, are also found within granulomas. Interferon-γ (IFN-γ) released by activated T cells causes macrophage transformation into epithelioid and giant cells. The granuloma is surrounded by a cuff of lymphocytes,

and the migration of fibroblasts results in increased collagen synthesis. Caseous necrotic areas may be present in the centre of a granuloma.

The nature of the damaging stimuli determines the type of granuloma formed. Inert particles (e.g. silica in the lungs) are predominantly surrounded by macrophages. Microorganisms such as *M. tuberculosis* induce a persistent delayed-type hypersensitivity (DTH) response, resulting in granuloma formation in the lung and possibly leading to cavitation (see p. 51). The granuloma formed is characterized by focal accumulation of lymphocytes and macrophages. The intensity of the DTH response is governed by the degree of hypersensitivity and not the antigenic load and in infection with *M. tuberculosis*, a DTH response is harmful to the host.

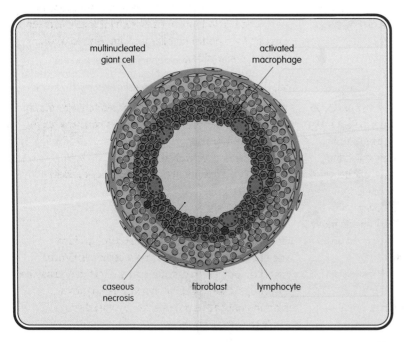

Fig. 4.7 A granuloma, showing typical focal accumulation of lymphocytes and macrophages around a central area of caseous necrosis.

Neutrophils are the main mediators of acute inflammation. Macrophages are central in chronic inflammation.

- What is inflammation?
- Summarize the underlying mechanisms, features, mediators, and possible outcomes of acute and chronic inflammation.
- Describe the role of adhesion molecules in acute inflammation.

HYPERSENSITIVITY MECHANISMS

The term hypersensitivity refers to exaggerated or inappropriate immune responses that cause tissue damage. The mechanisms involved are the same as those used to eliminate antigen under normal circumstances, but instead damage normal tissues. Hypersensitivity reactions have been classified into four types: I, II, III, and IV. Types I, II, and III are **antibody-mediated**; type IV is **cell-mediated**.

Type I hypersensitivity

In type I (or immediate) hypersensitivity, the antigen (allergen) induces a humoral IgE immune response. On first exposure to the allergen, an individual produces IgE specific for that allergen. IgE binds high-affinity FcεRs (receptors for the Fc portion of the IgE molecule), thus sensitizing mast cells and basophils. Upon subsequent exposures, cross-linking of membrane-bound IgE induces degranulation. Preformed and newly synthesized mediators are released. Their effects may be localized or systemic (see Fig. 3.6).

Examples of type I reactions include:
- Allergic rhinitis (hayfever).
- Allergic asthma.
- Systemic anaphylaxis due to penicillin administration.

Atopy is a genetic predisposition to produce IgE in response to many common, naturally occurring allergens. It has a prevalence of 10–30%. Atopic patients may suffer from multiple allergic disorders.

The **skin-prick test** is used to diagnose type I reactions: a number of allergens can be applied to adjacent areas of the skin of the forearm. A positive result is characterized by a wheal-and-flare reaction occurring within 15 minutes. Serum IgE levels (total and specific for a particular allergen) are used to assess type I hypersensitivity.

Type II hypersensitivity

Antibody specific for cell surface or extracellular matrix antigens is produced. Cell destruction can then result via several mechanisms:
- Complement activation.
- Antibody-dependent cell-mediated cytotoxicity (ADCC).
- Phagocytosis.

In some disorders, antibody against cell surface receptors stimulate or block the receptor. In Graves' disease, stimulating antibodies are directed against the thyrotropin (TSH) receptor. In myasthenia gravis, blocking antibodies are directed against the acetylcholine receptor.

49

Examples of type II reactions are:
- Incompatible blood transfusions.
- Haemolytic disease of the newborn.
- Autoimmune haemolytic anaemias.

Type III hypersensitivity

In type III (or immune-complex-mediated) hypersensitivity, antibody combines with soluble antigen. The resulting immune complexes are usually phagocytosed, but may persist depending on their size, and immune complex disease ensues (Fig. 4.8).

The immune complexes may be deposited in tissues near the site of antigen entry (*localized type III reaction*). This is demonstrated by the *Arthus reaction*. In an animal with high levels of appropriate

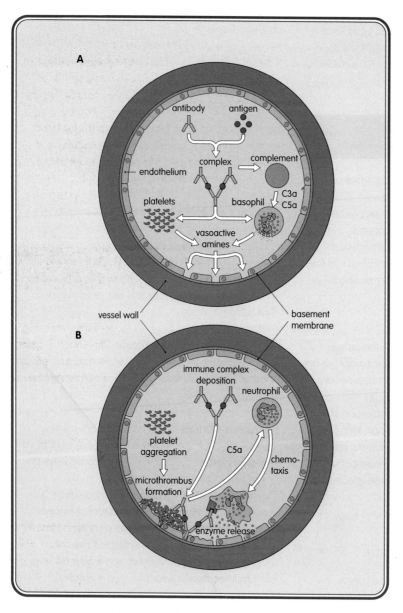

Fig. 4.8 (A) Antibody combines with soluble antigen to form immune complexes (ICs) which activate complement. The C3a and C5a generated induce degranulation of mast cells and basophils. Direct interaction of the ICs with Fc receptors on basophils and platelets also induces degranulation. The net effect is the release of vasoactive amines such as histamine and 5-HT, which cause endothelial cell retraction, increasing vascular permeability.
(B) The consequences of increased vascular permeability are twofold:
(1) ICs are deposited in the blood vessel wall and activate complement. The C5a generated is chemotactic for neutrophils, which migrate to the site of IC deposition and attempt to phagocytose the ICs but cannot as they are bound to the basement membrane. They release their lytic enzymes extracellularly ('frustrated phagocytosis').
(2) The exposed collagen of the basement membrane provides a site for platelet aggregation, which is facilitated by the interaction of platelets with the Fc portion of deposited ICs. This leads to microthrombus formation.

circulating antibody, an intradermal or subcutaneous injection of antigen produces localized immune complexes that activate complement and generate acute inflammation.

Localized type III reactions are exemplified by:
- Farmer's lung, which results from repeated inhalation of actinomycetes found in mouldy hay.
- Pigeon-fancier's disease, which results from repeated inhalation of antigens found in dried pigeon faeces.

If the immune complexes are formed in the blood, they circulate around the body and are deposited in the blood vessel walls of a number of tissues such as the kidneys and joints (*generalized type III reaction*). Historically, a generalized type III reaction was a complication of horse anti-tetanus serum administration. The symptoms were collectively called *serum sickness*.

Generalized type III reactions:
- Cause autoimmune diseases such as SLE.
- Occur in infectious diseases such as malaria and viral hepatitis.

Type IV hypersensitivity

Upon first contact with antigen, a subset of CD4$^+$ T helper (Th) cells is activated and clonally expanded (the *sensitization phase*). This takes 1–2 weeks, hence the alternative name of delayed-type hypersensitivity. Upon subsequent encounter with the same antigen, the sensitized Th cells secrete cytokines, which attract and activate macrophages (the *effector phase*). The activated macrophages have increased lytic and phagocytic ability and can destroy pathogens more effectively. The type IV reaction peaks at 48–72 hours after contact with the antigen. This is the time taken for the recruitment and activation of the macrophages. A type IV response is characterized by few antigen-specific T cells (less than 5% of the total) and many macrophages. Type IV reactions are important in the clearance of intracellular pathogens. However, if antigen persists, the response can be detrimental to the individual, as the lytic products of the activated macrophages can damage healthy tissues.

Examples of antigens that induce a type IV response are:
- Contact antigens such as nickel and poison ivy.
- Intracellular pathogens such as *Mycobacterium tuberculosis* and *Leishmania major*.

Skin testing is performed to detect type IV reactions. The tuberculin skin test can be used to determine whether a person has been exposed to *M. tuberculosis*. An intradermal injection of purified protein derivative (PPD) is given to the individual. Previous exposure to *M. tuberculosis* or bacille Calmette–Guérin (BCG) vaccination results in a positive response. This is apparent as a red, firm lesion at the injection site 48–72 hours after the injection. The lesion is due to the intense infiltration of macrophages at the injection site.

- Define hypersensitivity.
- Summarize the mechanisms underlying the four types of hypersensitivity reaction.
- Give examples of each of the four types of hypersensitivity reaction.

IMMUNE RESPONSE TO PATHOGENS

Viruses

Viruses are obligate intracellular parasites, requiring host enzymes for their replication. The immune system has to be able, firstly, to prevent infection, and secondly, once infection has occurred, to effectively eliminate an intracellular target.

Innate defences

Innate defences are important in the first few days of infection, when specific B and T cell clones have not developed. These include:
- Interferons (IFNs)—viral infection of the cell induces production of IFNs. These act on neighbouring uninfected cells and inhibit transcription and translation of viral proteins. In addition to its antiviral activity, IFN-γ activates macrophages and natural killer (NK) cells and enhances the adaptive immune response by upregulating expression of major histocompatibility complex (MHC) class I and II molecules.

- NK cells—these are cytotoxic for virus-infected cells and participate in antibody-dependent cell-mediated cytotoxicity (ADCC).

Adaptive immune response
Antibody-mediated immunity
Antibodies can bind to free virus and prevent its attachment and entry to a cell (neutralization of virus particles). For example, secreted IgA (sIgA), which is present in mucous secretions, can bind virus and prevent its attachment to mucosal epithelial cells.

Viral proteins are expressed on the surface of infected cells and act as targets for antibody recognition and binding:

- Antibodies can opsonize infected cells.
- Virus-infected cells can be destroyed by ADCC and complement activation.

Responses directed against free virus are considered to be the most important *in vivo*, and antibodies are therefore important early in the course of infection by preventing spread of virus between cells.

Cell-mediated immunity
Once infection has been established, the following cell-mediated mechanisms are important in eliminating virus:

- Viral peptides presented on the cell surface in association with class I MHC molecules are recognized by cytotoxic CD8+ T cells, which can destroy the infected cell.
- CD4+ T cell help is required for the generation of the antibody and cytotoxic T cell responses, and the recruitment and activation of macrophages.

Bacteria
Different mechanisms operate depending on whether the bacteria are extracellular or intracellular.

Innate defences
Extracellular bacteria
Bacteria with appropriate carbohydrates on their surface can bind and activate mannan-binding protein, thus activating complement via the lectin pathway. Some bacteria can activate complement via the alternative pathway. Activated complement products play a role in the elimination of bacteria, especially C3b (an opsonin), C3a and C5a (anaphylatoxins that recruit leucocytes), and the membrane-attack complex (MAC), which can perforate the outer lipid bilayer of Gram-negative bacteria. Most bacteria are killed by phagocytic cells, and bacterial binding to phagocytes is enhanced by C3b.

Intracellular bacteria
Like viruses, intracellular bacteria can activate NK cells, which produce IFN-γ, a potent activating factor for macrophages.

Adaptive immune response
Extracellular bacteria: antibody-mediated immunity
This is the principal defence against extracellular bacteria:

- sIgA binds to bacteria and prevents their binding to epithelial cells.
- Antibody neutralizes bacterial toxins.
- Antibody activates complement—this is the most important role of antibody in defence against bacteria (the resultant C3b acts as an opsonin).
- Antibody acts as an opsonin.

Extracellular bacteria: cell-mediated immunity
Bacterial antigens are processed and presented—in conjunction with class II MHC molecules on the surface of antigen-presenting cells (APCs)—to CD4+ T cells:

- CD4+ T cells secrete IFN-γ, which activates macrophages.
- CD4+ T cell help is required for the generation of the antibody response.

Intracellular bacteria
Cell-mediated immunity is very important in defence against intracellular bacterial infections such as those caused by *M. tuberculosis*:

- Cytokines released by CD4+ T cells activate macrophages, which attempt to phagocytose the bacteria. If the organisms persist, tissue damage can occur (type IV hypersensitivity reaction; see p. 51).
- CD8+ T cells recognize antigens presented in conjunction with class I MHC molecules on the surface of infected cells and lyse these cells.

Protozoa
Protozoa are larger than bacteria and viruses and have more complex life cycles, with several different stages. They therefore present the immune system with a variety of options. Protozoan infection is often chronic, as the immune system is not very efficient at dealing with these organisms.

Innate defences

These include phagocytosis by macrophages, monocytes, and neutrophils, which can be enhanced by antibody or complement components acting as opsonins.

Adaptive immune response
Antibody-mediated immunity

This is important in counteracting extracellular, circulating forms of protozoa (neutralizing antibodies prevent attachment and spread of protozoa).

Cell-mediated immunity

This is important in combatting the intracellular stages of protozoan infection. Both CD4+ and CD8+ T cells are important:

- The subset of CD4+ T cells activated is thought to determine whether the immune response is protective or not, depending on the secreted cytokine profile.
- Cytotoxic CD8+ T cells are important in destroying protozoa that replicate within cells, e.g. the sporozoite stage of *Plasmodium falciparum*.

Evasion of the immune response

Pathogens may evade the immune response in a number of ways. For example:

- Antigenic shift and drift are mechanisms of antigenic variation that are exhibited by the influenza virus.
- Encapsulated bacteria, e.g. *Streptococcus pneumoniae*, are more resistant to phagocytosis.
- Mycobacteria inhibit phagolysosome formation.
- The variant surface glycoprotein coat of trypanosomes is subject to antigenic shift.

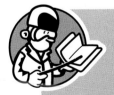

- **List the innate and adaptive defence mechanisms used against viruses, bacteria, and protozoa.**
- **Give examples of how organisms can evade the immune response.**

AUTOIMMUNITY AND IMMUNE DISEASE

Autoimmunity is a state in which the body exhibits immunological reactivity to itself.

'Self-tolerance' is the generic term given to the mechanisms by which T and B cells are prevented from responding to self.

Mechanisms of self-tolerance
Tolerance induced by early clonal deletion

Negative selection causes the elimination of T cells (in the thymus) and B cells (in the bone marrow) that are self-reactive.

Tolerance due to clonal anergy

Non-deleted self-reactive T cells may undergo clonal anergy via a number of mechanisms:

- T cell activation in the absence of a variable co-stimulatory signal (e.g. IL-1 production) leads to the selective inhibition of IL-2 production, preventing autocrine 'IL-2–IL-2-receptor-mediated' activation.
- Downregulation of the T cell receptor (TCR) on CD8+ T cells may lead to impaired recognition of self-antigen presented by class I MHC molecules.
- Thymic epithelial cells may also render developing T cells anergic.

Tolerance due to the selective migration of lymphocytes

Antigens associated with peripheral tissues, especially those sequestered behind anatomical barriers in 'immunologically privileged' sites, may not come into contact with the T cell repertoire: for example, lens protein of the eye. Tolerance is therefore unnecessary.

T-cell-mediated suppression

This includes the following:

- IL-10 released by Th2 cells may impair the co-stimulatory signal provided by APCs, rendering Th1 cells anergic.
- A lack of T cell help may render autoreactive B cells anergic.
- Proliferation of autoreactive T cells may be prevented by the absorption of essential cytokines by the 'target' cell.

The mechanisms described previously, contribute to self-tolerance, but may break down via a number of processes.

Breakdown of self-tolerance
Molecular mimicry
Certain bacteria and viruses possess antigens that resemble sequestered host-cell components, and infection with these may generate an immune response against self. The MHC haplotype may influence susceptibility to this form of autoimmunity. Viruses may also resemble non-sequestered antigens; e.g. cross-reactivity between heart muscle and streptococcal antigens, leading to rheumatic fever. This is short-lived and reversible.

Release of sequestered antigens
Certain antigens are not seen by the developing immune system, and exposure after development may lead to self-reactivity. Tissue trauma may release previously sequestered antigen into the circulation, and an immune response may consequently develop.

Cytokine imbalance, dysfunction of immune regulation, and inappropriate MHC expression
Inappropriate T cell activation results in the upregulation of MHC class II molecules and may result in activation of autoreactive T cells. Healthy β cells of the islets of Langerhans have been shown to express low levels of class I and II MHC molecules, whilst cells in individuals with insulin-dependent diabetes mellitus (IDDM) express high levels of both.

Polyclonal B cell activation
Viruses such as Epstein–Barr virus and cytomegalovirus may cause the non-specific activation and proliferation of numerous clones of B cells, resulting in the production of autoantibodies.

It is important to remember that the causes of autoimmunity are multifactorial and a defect in some or all of the regulatory mechanisms are required before an autoimmune disease develops.

Autoimmune disease
The types of autoantigens involved in autoimmune responses are listed in Fig. 4.9.

Pathogenic mechanisms involved in autoimmunity
Antibody-mediated (type II hypersensitivity reactions)
These include:
- Neutralization—e.g. in pernicious anaemia, antibodies to intrinsic factor block uptake of vitamin B_{12}.
- Complement fixation—e.g. C3b binding in Goodpasture's syndrome.
- Opsonization—e.g. red blood cells and antibodies in autoimmune haemolytic anaemia.
- ADCC—e.g. in Hashimoto's thyroiditis.

Immune-complex-mediated (type III hypersensitivity reactions)
Circulating antigen, antibody, and complement complexes can be taken up by phagocytic cells (e.g. polymorphs), causing release of vasoactive peptides and enzymes. Immune complexes localize in joints and kidneys in, for example, rheumatoid arthritis.

Cell-mediated (type IV hypersensitivity reactions)
These comprise autoimmune T cell responses, usually by T helper and T cytotoxic cells.

Autoantigens involved in autoimmune responses	
Type	**Example**
plasma proteins	thyroglobulin (Tg) in Hashimoto's thyroiditis; IgG in rheumatoid arthritis
functional membrane receptors	TSH receptor on thyroid cells in Graves' disease; acetylcholine receptors in myasthenia gravis
cell membrane antigens	RBC in autoimmune haemolytic anaemia, anti-Rhesus antibodies; platelets in idiopathic thrombocytopenic purpura
extracellular antigens (e.g. basement membranes)	antibodies to basement membrane of lungs and kidney in Goodpasture's syndrome
intracellular antigens	single-stranded and double-stranded DNA and mitochondria in many mixed connective tissue diseases, e.g. SLE and primary biliary cirrhosis

Fig. 4.9 Types of autoantigens involved in autoimmune responses.

Possible aetiologies of autoimmunity

These include:

- Genetic—many autoimmune diseases are familial, but environmental factors also play an important role. Among patients with Graves' disease, 50% have a positive family history, and 50% of monozygotic twins develop the disease, but the concordance is only 5% in dizygotic twins.
- HLA associations—e.g. HLA-DR4 in rheumatoid arthritis. However, a certain HLA haplotype does not automatically result in the development of an autoimmune disease: e.g. 95% of patients with ankylosing spondylitis have HLA-B27, but only 5% of the population with HLA-B27 have ankylosing spondylitis.

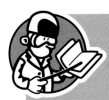

- ○ **Describe the mechanisms by which self-tolerance is maintained.**
- ○ **How might these mechanisms break down?**
- ○ **List the various types of autoantigen that form the focus of an autoimmune disease.**

IMMUNIZATION

Immunity can be achieved by passive or active immunization (Fig. 4.10).

Active immunization

Active immunization usually requires contact with the antigens of the microorganism, either through natural infection or by vaccination. Individuals exhibit a primary immune response, with clonal expansion of B and T cells and formation of memory cells. Consequently, subsequent exposure to the same antigen will induce a secondary immune response.

Vaccination is a form of active immunization. It aims to induce specific immunity to a particular pathogen so that on re-exposure to that pathogen, a rapid, protective immune response will be evoked.

An ideal vaccine is:

- *Safe*, with minimal side effects and free of contaminating substances.
- *Immunogenic*, activating the required branches of the immune system, inducing long-lasting local and systemic immunity.
- *Heat stable*, as it is difficult to maintain the cold chain in tropical countries.
- *Inexpensive*, an important consideration, especially in Third World countries.

Comparison of passive and active immunization		
	Passive immunization	**Active immunization**
features	preformed immunoglobulins transferred to individual	contact with antigen induces adpative immune response
advantages	large amounts of antibody available immediately	long-lived immunity induced
disadvantages	short lifespan of antibodies; risk of anti-isotype reaction if antibodies raised in another species, e.g. serum sickness (see p. 51); risk of antiallotype reaction if human immunoglobulin used	takes some time to develop immunity
examples	transfer of maternal antibody across placenta to fetus; administration of human anti-tetanus toxin immunoglobulin	natural exposure to a pathogen; vaccination

Fig. 4.10 Comparison of passive and active immunization.

The types of vaccine in current use are listed in Fig. 4.11. The two main types, live and killed, are compared in Fig. 4.12. The routine immunization schedule used in the United Kingdom is shown in Fig. 4.13.

Adjuvants are substances that non-specifically heighten the immune response. Examples include aluminium salts and *Bordetella pertussis*.

A small proportion of individuals receiving vaccination will not respond adequately. This does not matter if the the majority of the population is immune to the organism, as the non-responders are unlikely to come into contact with infected individuals (*herd immunity*).

Passive immunization

Passive immunization involves the transfer of preformed immunoglobulins to an individual. Contact with antigen is not required. Passive immunization is used if an individual is exposed to an organism to which he or she does not have active immunity.

Bacterial

Antitoxins, i.e. antibodies directed against toxins, are used in the treatment of:

- Tetanus (tetanus toxoid is given at the same time to inadequately immunized individuals).
- Diphtheria.
- Botulism.

Viral

Specific immunoglobulin preparations are used after exposure to:

- Rabies (killed vaccine may be administered at the same time).

> Vaccination is an important topic that will crop up not only in your immunology exam but also in your clinical studies. Be able to reproduce Figs 4.11–4.13 as you are likely to be examined on these in the short-answer section of the paper.

Different types of vaccine in use today		
Vaccine	**Features**	**Examples**
live attenuated	attenuation achieved by repeated subculture of organism on artificial media or by serial passage in animals; immunogenicity is retained, but virulence is significantly diminished	oral polio (OPV, Sabin), BCG (bacille Calmette-Guérin)
killed	intact organisms killed by exposure to heat or chemicals, e.g. formalin	polio (Salk), pertussis
subunit	purified, protective immunity-inducing antigenic components; often surface antigens (most accessible to immune system)	influenza, pneumococcal vaccine
recombinant	genes encoding epitopes that elicit protective immune response inserted into prokaryotic or eukaryotic cells; large quantities of vaccine rapidly produced	surface antigen of hepatitis B (hepBsAg), which is produced in yeast cells
toxoids	bacterial toxins inactivated by exposure to heat or chemicals	diphtheria, tetanus
conjugates	polysaccharide antigen linked to protein carrier, which enhances immunogenicity	Hib (*Haemophilus influenzae* type b) —a type b capsular polysaccharide linked to e.g. tetanus toxoid

Fig. 4.11 Different types of vaccine in use today.

- Hepatitis B (recombinant vaccine may be administered at the same time).
- Varicella zoster (to immunocompromised individuals).

Human normal immunoglobulin can be administered after exposure to:

- Hepatitis A.
- Measles (to immunocompromised individuals).

Features of live versus killed vaccines		
Feature	**Live vaccine**	**Killed vaccine**
level of immunity induced	high—organisms replicate in host (mimicking natural infection), producing long-lasting antigenic challenge	low—organisms do not replicate, producing short-lived stimulus
dose required	usually single	several booster doses
cell-mediated response	good—replication in host cells means antigens are processed and presented with MHC molecules	poor
local immunity	good, e.g. OPV	poor
cost	cheaper than killed vaccines	more expensive to produce and administer than live attenuated vaccines
reversion to virulence	possible but rare (not safe during immunosuppression or pregnancy)	no (therefore safe for immunocompromised and pregnant patients)
stability	heat labile	heat stable
risk of contamination	possible—by another virus present in the cell culture used to prepare vaccine	n/a

Fig. 4.12 Features of live versus killed vaccines.

Routine immunization schedule in the UK	
Vaccine	**Age**
D/T/P (diphtheria, tetanus, pertussis), OPV, and Hib	three doses—at 2, 3, and 4 months
MMR (measles, mumps, rubella)	12–18 months
booster D/T and OPV	4–5 years
BCG	10–14 years or infancy
booster tetanus and OPV	15–18 years

Fig. 4.13 The routine immunization schedule used in the UK.

- Summarize the concepts of active and passive immunization, and their uses, advantages, and disadvantages.
- Describe the concept of herd immunity.
- What different types of vaccine are available? Give examples of each.
- Compare and contrast live and killed vaccines.
- Describe the routine immunization schedule in the UK.

TRANSPLANTATION

The following definitions are important:
- Autologous graft—a graft from one part of the body to another, e.g. a skin graft.
- Syngeneic graft—a graft between genetically identical individuals, e.g. monozygotic twins.
- Allogeneic graft—a graft between individuals of the same species (a common clinical situation).
- Xenogeneic graft—a graft between individuals of different species.

Transplant rejection

Unless the donor and recipient are immunologically identical, a rejection response will occur. The success of the transplant relies on minimizing this response. Rejection occurs because the recipient's immune system recognizes and responds to foreign antigens expressed by the graft. The most important graft antigens responsible for an immune response in the recipient are the MHC molecules (see Chapter 3).

T cells are essential for rejection: native APCs process and present graft antigens to the recipient's CD4+ T cells. A far more powerful stimulus, however, is that provided by donor APCs present in the graft. Foreign MHC molecules expressed by them can activate T cells directly. Activated CD4+ T cells release cytokines, which activate several cell types—including cytotoxic T cells, macrophages, B cells, and vascular endothelial cells—and upregulate MHC expression, leading to a rejection response. Even when the donor and recipient are genetically identical at the MHC loci, graft rejection can occur due to differences at other loci which encode *minor histocompatibility antigens*.

There are four types of graft rejection (Fig. 4.14):
- Hyperacute.
- Acute vascular.
- Acute cellular.
- Chronic.

Hyperacute rejection

In this type of rejection, pre-existing antidonor antibodies induced by previous immunization episodes (e.g. blood transfusions) bind molecules on the blood vessel endothelial cells. The complement and clotting cascades are activated. There is intense neutrophil infiltration, and platelet aggregation causes thrombus formation, which blocks blood vessels, leading to ischaemia and necrosis of the graft.

Acute vascular rejection

This is similar to hyperacute rejection, but the recipient initially has a lower titre of antidonor antibodies, so a cross-match of donor cells and recipient serum may be negative. For this reason, old serum samples, which have ideally been collected after every immunization episode, should be tested. If a match with an old serum sample is positive, even if that with the current sample is negative, there is a risk of acute vascular rejection.

Patterns of graft rejection		
Type of rejection	**Mechanism of rejection**	**Prevention** (e.g. for kidney transplant)
hyperacute (minutes to hours)	pre-existing antidonor antibodies	perform cross-match of donor cells and recipient's serum; check for ABO incompatibility
acute vascular (1–2 days)	pre-existing antidonor antibodies	as for hyperacute rejection, but old serum samples should also be checked
acute cellular (days to weeks)	T cell-mediated	HLA matching of donor and recipient; antirejection therapy
chronic (months to years)	unclear	HLA matching beneficial

Fig. 4.14 Patterns of graft rejection.

Acute cellular rejection

This is mediated by T cells and would occur in all allogeneic grafts unless prevented by antirejection therapy. If the recipient has T cells sensitized to graft antigens before receiving the graft, rejection is accelerated (second-set or 'white graft' rejection).

Chronic

The mechanisms underlying chronic rejection are unclear. Some possibilities include deposition of antibodies and immune complexes on the endothelial cells, low grade cell-mediated rejection, recurrence of the original disease in the graft, and viral infection of the graft.

Strategies for preventing rejection

The rejection response can be reduced by MHC matching of the donor and recipient and by instituting antirejection therapy.

Matching

The ideal match is that between monozygotic twins. In all other situations, there will be some genetic disparity between donor and recipient. The aim of matching is to minimize genetic differences between donor and recipient, in particular those at MHC loci.

Antirejection therapy

The following drugs can be used to immunosuppress the recipient:
- Steroids—these are anti-inflammatory.
- Cyclosporin—inhibits IL-2 secretion by Th cells and downregulates IL-2 receptor expression by lymphocytes, inhibiting their activation.
- Azathioprine—an antiproliferative drug.

The disadvantage of such non-specific therapy is that the recipient is at increased risk of opportunistic infections (e.g. cytomegalovirus) and certain malignancies. Newer, more selective agents are being developed, including anti-CD3 monoclonal antibodies.

The types of transplantation performed today are summarized in Fig. 4.15.

- Why are transplanted organs rejected?
- What are the four types of rejection and how may they be prevented?
- Describe the types of transplantation performed today.

Types of transplantation performed today	
Transplant	**Notes**
kidney	live/cadaveric donor; the fewer the MHC mismatches, the greater the success rate; ABO compatibility required
heart	matching beneficial, but usually not enough time
liver	no evidence that matching affects graft survival, and usually not enough time; rejection less aggressive than for other organs
skin graft	matching not required; allografts used for temporary protection of burns patients; host cells replace donor cells after few weeks
corneal graft	matching usually not required; if graft is vascularized (5% of cases) and rejection occurs, matching for class II needed before further grafting
bone marrow	host-versus-graft (HVG) or graft-versus-host (GVH) responses possible; minimize by matching, anti-rejection therapy, total body irradiation before transplantation (HVG), depletion of T cells (which mediate GVH response) with monoclonal antibody plus complement

Fig. 4.15 Types of transplantation performed today.

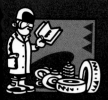

5. Red Blood Cells and Haemoglobin

Structure

Erythrocytes are mature red cells (Fig. 5.1). They are not nucleated and contain no organelles.

Morphology is routinely examined on Romanovsky-stained blood smears: erythrocytes stain pink because of their high haemoglobin content, with a pale-staining centre due to their biconcave discoid shape. Their average lifespan is 120 days, during which they travel 300 miles through the circulation. An erythrocyte has an average diameter of 7.2 μm and yet it passes through vessels of the microcirculation that have a minimum diameter of 3 μm. This task requires flexibility and deformability. As a biconcave disc, the erythrocyte has a surface area that is 20–30% greater than that of a sphere of the same volume, facilitating gas exchange, the primary function of the erythrocyte.

Function

The erythrocyte carries oxygen from the lungs to the tissues, and carbon dioxide from the tissues to the lungs.

Oxygen carriage

The solubility of oxygen in the blood is 0.03 mL/L blood per mmHg O_2. The body's resting requirement of O_2, however, is 250 mL/min. If the body was to rely on dissolved oxygen alone, an impossibly high ventilation rate would be required to fulfil its oxygen requirement. Each erythrocyte contains 640 million molecules of haemoglobin, an oxygen-carrying pigment that gives blood its red colour. Over 99% of the oxygen contained in blood is carried by haemoglobin. The oxygen content of the blood depends on three factors:

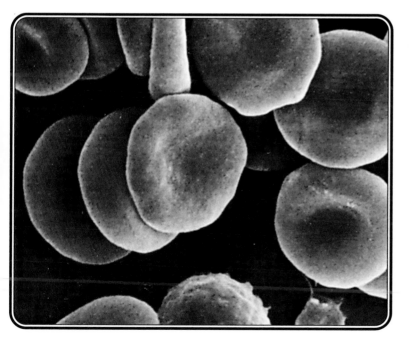

Fig. 5.1 Scanning electron micrograph of red blood cells (Courtesy of Dr Trevor Gray).

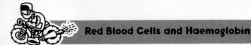
- The concentration of haemoglobin.
- The affinity of haemoglobin for oxygen (see p. 70).
- The amount of dissolved oxygen (this is small).

Carbon dioxide carriage

This is carried in three forms (Fig. 5.2):

- Approximately 90% as bicarbonate.

- Approximately 5% in the form of carbamino compounds (CO_2 combines with the amino groups of plasma proteins and also haemoglobin).
- Approximately 5% in physical solution (CO_2 is over 20 times more soluble in blood than is O_2).

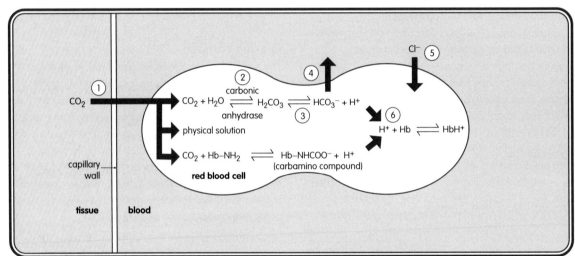

Fig. 5.2 Carriage of carbon dioxide in the blood. Only the intracellular pathways are shown. Similar mechanisms operate in the plasma. (1) CO_2 passes down its partial pressure gradient from tissue to blood. (2) It combines with water to form carbonic acid (H_2CO_3). The enzyme carbonic anhydrase (present in red cells) accelerates this step, which is otherwise slow in plasma. (3) H_2CO_3 is a weak acid and dissociates into protons (H^+) and bicarbonate ions (HCO_3^-). (4) Bicarbonate ions are produced mainly in the red cells rather than the plasma and so a concentration gradient is set up, promoting diffusion of HCO_3^- out of the cell into the plasma. (5) Due to the exit of HCO_3^-, the inside of the cell is positively charged relative to plasma. Chloride ions (Cl^-) pass from the plasma into the red cells to maintain electroneutrality. This HCO_3^-/Cl^- exchange is called the *chloride shift*. (6) Protons are generated as a result of two processes: the formation of bicarbonate ions and the dissociation of carbamino compounds. The red cell membrane is impermeable to protons, which must therefore be buffered. Intracellularly, this function is fulfilled by the imidazole groups of the haemoglobin molecule (extracellularly, the plasma proteins fulfil this function).

 Carbon dioxide carriage is a common topic for short-answer questions. Be able to sketch Fig. 5.2 and explain each step.

- Describe how the structure of the erythrocyte is related to its function.
- Summarize how carbon dioxide is carried in the blood.

ERYTHROPOIESIS

Erythropoiesis is the production of red blood cells [cf. haemopoiesis—the production of red and white blood cells (see Chapter 1)].

A steady-state system operates in which the production of new blood cells balances removal of mature cells in the spleen.

Sequence of erythropoiesis

Erythropoiesis occurs in erythroblastic islands within the bone marrow. These contain macrophages, which supply iron to the surrounding erythroid progenitor cells. The entire sequence (from stem cell to erythrocyte) takes approximately 1 week. Maturation is characterized by the following stages:
- Pronormoblast.
- Early, intermediate, and late normoblasts.
- Reticulocyte.
- Erythrocyte.

In the following cell descriptions, the appearance is that seen with the routine Romanovsky stain, unless otherwise specified.

Pronormoblast

The pronormoblast is the earliest recognizable erythroid cell in the bone marrow. It is a large cell that has a small amount of basophilic (blue) cytoplasm, a large nucleus with finely dispersed nuclear chromatin, and lots of organelles. It does not contain haemoglobin.

Early, intermediate, and late normoblasts

These cells display progressive changes in cell appearance:
- Decrease in cell size.
- Decrease in nuclear size.
- Increased condensation of chromatin.
- Increase in cytoplasmic volume:nuclear volume ratio.
- Decreased basophilia due to a decrease in ribosomal RNA (stains blue).
- Increased eosinophilia due to an increase in haemoglobin (stains pink) synthesis.

Reticulocyte

A pyknotic (condensed) nucleus is extruded from the late normoblast, and an anucleate reticulocyte is released from the bone marrow. The latter contains some organelles, including ribosomes, and can therefore continue haemoglobin synthesis (20–30% of total haemoglobin synthesis occurs at this stage). Reticulocytes circulate in peripheral blood for 1–2 days before maturing and account for 1–2% of the red cell count. They are difficult to distinguish from mature erythrocytes on a routine stain, but, if incubated with the dye brilliant cresyl blue (supravital staining), the RNA in ribosomes precipitates and appears blue.

Erythrocyte

The mature erythrocyte appears pink and contains no organelles.

Following severe erythrocyte depletion, e.g. due to haemolysis, the rate of erythropoiesis in the bone marrow increases. Nucleated precursors and an increased number of reticulocytes appear in the peripheral blood.

Ineffective erythropoiesis

Each pronormoblast can potentially give rise to 16 erythrocytes, but some normoblasts fail to develop and are phagocytosed by bone marrow macrophages. In a healthy individual, the amount of ineffective erythropoiesis is small.

Regulation of erythropoiesis

The principal factor involved in regulation of this pathway is a hormone called erythropoietin (EPO), which is secreted by:
- Endothelial cells of the peritubular capillaries in the renal cortex (85%).
- Kupffer cells and hepatocytes in the liver (15%).

Increased erythropoietin drive

The major stimulus for secretion is *hypoxia*. This can be caused by any factor that gives rise to decreased oxygen transport to tissues relative to tissue demand and is not necessarily due to a decrease in red cell number (Fig. 5.3).

Decreased erythropoietin drive

Long standing renal disease—caused by a decrease in, or a complete loss of, renal mass, e.g. following

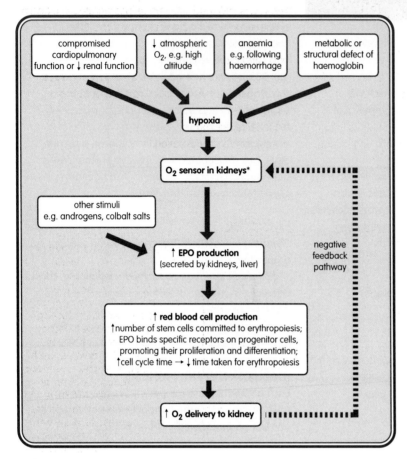

Fig. 5.3 Regulation of erythropoietin (EPO) production. A chronic state of increased EPO drive can result in expansion of erythropoiesis into fatty marrow and extramedullary sites. *The oxygen sensor in the kidneys is thought to be a haem protein that stimulates or inhibits transcription of the EPO gene, depending on its state of oxygenation.

chronic renal failure—or bilateral nephrectomy can lead to decreased production of EPO, resulting in anaemia. Recombinant EPO, produced in animal cells, is currently in clinical use. Indications for its use include:
- Anaemia due to renal failure.
- Autologous blood transfusions.
- After chemotherapy or bone marrow transplantation.
- Anaemia of chronic disease.

Erythropoiesis is also regulated by the availability of red cell components, most importantly iron, folic acid, and vitamin B_{12}.

○ **Describe the sequence of erythropoiesis.**
○ **What is ineffective erythropoiesis?**
○ **What is the role of erythropoietin in the regulation of erythropoiesis?**

IRON AND HAEM METABOLISM

Iron

Uptake and excretion of iron

Normal uptake and excretion of iron is illustrated in Fig. 5.4.

The rate of transfer of iron from epithelial cells to plasma responds to iron requirements, e.g. it is high when stores are low or the rate of erythropoiesis is high. The control mechanism, however, is poorly understood.

Free iron is toxic and is therefore incorporated into haem or bound to protein within the body (Fig. 5.5).

Iron overload

There is no mechanism for the excretion of excess iron. Consequently, iron overload can occur as a result of its:

- Increased absorption.
- Parenteral administration.

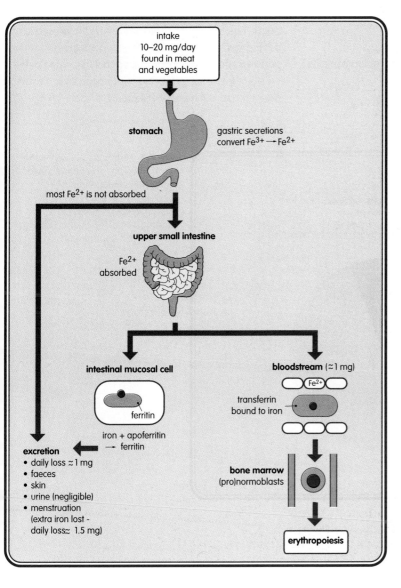

Fig. 5.4 Iron metabolism. Iron is converted in the stomach from Fe^{3+} to Fe^{2+}, which is more readily absorbed. Fe^{2+} is absorbed in the duodenum and jejunum by an active process. This is facilitated by ascorbic acid and other reducing agents, which promote the ferrous form, and inhibited by phytates, tannic acid, and tetracycline which form in soluble complexes with iron. In intestinal mucosal cells, some iron binds apoferritin, to form ferritin, a storage compound: the cells are ultimately shed into the gut lumen. The remaining iron is transported to the blood, where it binds transferrin, a transport protein: the bound iron is transported to storage compartments and to the bone marrow, where it is used for erythropoiesis. Iron that is not absorbed in the gut and that which is contained in shed mucosal cells is eliminated in the faeces. Some is lost in shed skin cells and in the urine.

Increased absorption

This can result from the following:

- Primary/hereditary haemochromatosis—an autosomal recessive disorder characterized by excessive intestinal absorption of iron. All other disorders characterized by iron overload are referred to as secondary haemochromatosis or haemosiderosis.
- Erythroid hyperplasia secondary to ineffective erythropoiesis or haemolysis, e.g. thalassaemia syndromes.
- Dietary excess (rare).
- Inappropriate oral therapy.

Parenteral administration

Examples include:

- Multiple blood transfusions (1 unit of blood contains 250 mg of iron).
- Inappropriate parenteral iron therapy.

Treatment

It is important to start therapy as soon as possible in order to prevent irreversible organ damage. Options include:

- Dietary advice (decrease intake of iron, increase intake of natural chelators).
- Venesection.
- Chelation therapy—desferrioxamine is an iron-chelating agent that is administered subcutaneously. Its cost, however, precludes its use in countries where the thalassaemia syndromes are prevalent.

Haem

Haem belongs to a family of compounds known as the porphyrins, which are characterized by the presence of a tetrapyrrole ring. Haem is an iron-containing porphyrin derivative, the iron atom being located at the centre of the tetrapyrrole ring of protoporphyrin IX. The haem group is the prosthetic group of haemoglobin

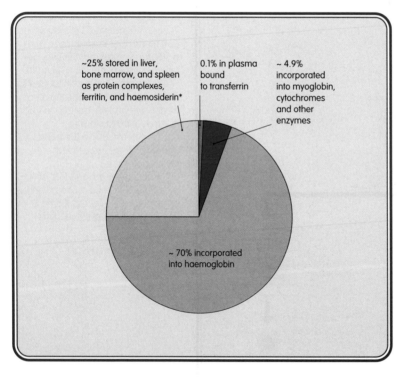

Fig. 5.5 Distribution of iron in the body. *Ferritin is a water-soluble compound, consisting of protein and iron, whereas haemosiderin is insoluble and consists of aggregates of ferritin that have lost their protein component.

~25% stored in liver, bone marrow, and spleen as protein complexes, ferritin, and haemosiderin*

0.1% in plasma bound to transferrin

~ 4.9% incorporated into myoglobin, cytochromes and other enzymes

~ 70% incorporated into haemoglobin

and is responsible for its oxygen-binding properties. Biosynthesis of haem and its disorders are discussed in *Crash Course: Metabolism and Nutrition*. Degradation occurs in the macrophages of the spleen, bone marrow, and liver (Fig. 5.6).

This process is speeded up in haemolytic anaemias (red cells have a shortened lifespan and are destroyed at an accelerated rate). This increased red cell destruction leads to anaemia, which stimulates increased EPO production, leading to

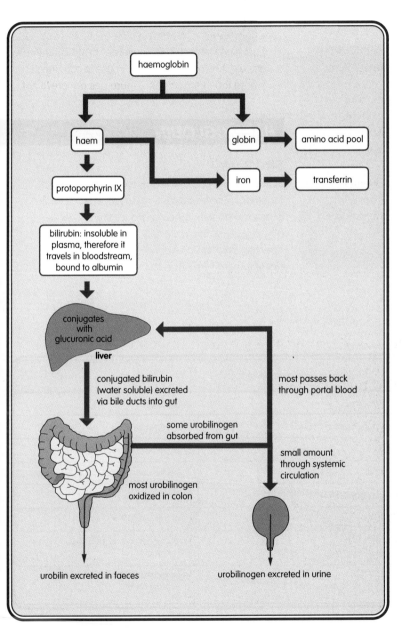

Fig. 5.6 Degradation of haemoglobin.

compensatory erythropoiesis. The clinical features of these conditions result from the increased red cell destruction and the compensatory increase in red cell production (Fig. 5.7).

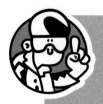

You can work out the clinical features of haemolytic anaemias by understanding the pathway of haem degradation.

○ **Describe the uptake, distribution, and excretion of iron.**
○ **Summarize the causes and consequences of iron overload.**
○ **Summarize the pathway of haem breakdown and describe how this relates to the clinical features of haemolytic anaemias.**

HAEMOGLOBIN

Structure

Haemoglobin consists of four globin chains held together by non-covalent interactions. Each chain is associated with a haem group, the oxygen-binding site of the molecule. Different types of haemoglobin are present at different stages of development (Fig 5.8).

Clinical features of haemolytic anaemias		
	Clinical feature	**Explanation**
features due to increased red cell destruction (see Fig. 5.6)	pallor of mucous membranes	↓ haemoglobin
	jaundice	↑ serum bilirubin (mainly unconjugated)
	urine darkens on standing	↑ urobilinogen, which is oxidized to urobilin
	pigment gall stones (i.e. consisting of bilirubin)	↑ bilirubin in bile
	splenomegaly	↑ red cell destruction
features due to increased red cell production (compensatory)	folate deficiency	↑ requirement due to increased red blood cell production
	bone deformities	erythroid hyperplasia causes expansion of marrow cavities

Fig. 5.7 Clinical features of haemolytic anaemias.

The structure of HbA

Adult haemoglobin (HbA) contains two α- and two β-chains, which are arranged as two dimers, written 2(αβ)—(Fig 5.9). The haem pocket is a hydrophobic crevice in each globin chain, wherein the haem molecule sits. Proximal histidine molecules in the

Haemoglobin during development		
Haemoglobin (Hb)	**Globin chains**	**Notes**
embryonic Hb		
Hb Gower I	$\zeta_2\epsilon_2$	ζ- and ε-chains synthesized soon after conception; later, ζ is replaced by α, and ε by γ and then β
Hb Gower II	$\alpha_2\epsilon_2$	
Hb Portland	$\zeta_2\gamma_2$	
fetal Hb		
HbF	$\alpha_2\gamma_2$	main Hb during later two-thirds of fetal life and in newborn; higher affinity for O_2 than HbA; < 1% Hb in adults
adult Hb		
HbA	$\alpha_2\beta_2$	principal Hb in adults; molecular weight 68 000 D
HbA$_2$	$\alpha_2\delta_2$	~2% of total Hb in adults

Fig. 5.8 Types of haemoglobin present during different stages of development.

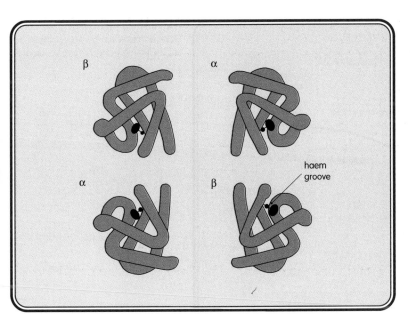

Fig. 5.9 Structure of adult haemoglobin (HbA). The α-chain comprises 141 amino acids; the β-chain, 146 amino acids.

haem pocket bind to the iron portion of the haem molecule, and distal histidine molecules help stabilize Fe^{2+}. The haem pocket allows the haem molecule to bind O_2 whilst protecting the iron atom from oxidation.

The other major haemoprotein in humans is myoglobin, which consists of a single chain associated with a haem group. It is found principally in muscle, where it provides an oxygen reserve. The four haemoglobin subunits are structurally similar to myoglobin. Certain functional features are unique to haemoglobin: this is due to the interaction between the globin subunits in the molecule.

Physiological properties of haemoglobin

Each haemoglobin molecule can bind four molecules of oxygen, one at each haem site. Deoxyhaemoglobin—taut (T-) haemoglobin—is characterized by a relatively large number of ionic and hydrogen bonds between the $\alpha\beta$ dimers, which restrict the movement of the globin chains. Upon binding of O_2, these bonds are broken and the dimers can move more freely relative to each other, allowing oxygen release. This is the relaxed (R-) form of the molecule.

The oxygen dissociation curve is a plot of partial pressure of oxygen (x axis) against oxygen saturation (y axis) (Fig 5.10).

The haemoglobin curve is sigmoidal in shape because of the cooperative binding of oxygen to haemoglobin: the binding of O_2 to one haem group enhances binding at the other haem sites on the same haemoglobin molecule. Conversely, unloading of O_2 at one haem group facilitates unloading at the other haem sites. In comparison, the myoglobin curve is hyperbolic in shape as myoglobin does not release oxygen until the partial pressure of O_2 falls to very low levels. This is because myoglobin does not exhibit cooperative binding.

Changes in CO_2, H^+, 2,3-diphosphoglycerate (2,3-DPG), and temperature, shift the position of the haemoglobin curve but do not generally alter its shape (Fig. 5.10). Binding of oxygen to myoglobin is not altered

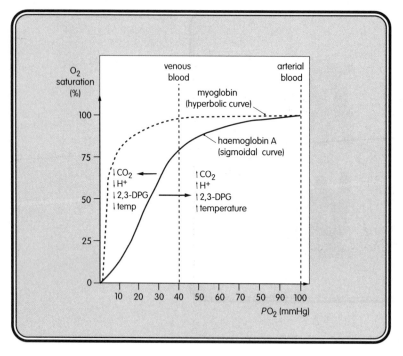

Fig. 5.10 Oxygen dissociation curve for haemoglobin and myoglobin. (2,3-DPG, 2,3-diphosphoglycerate.)

by these factors. CO_2, H^+, and 2,3-DPG bind to and stabilize deoxyhaemoglobin, favouring unloading of oxygen. The shift of the curve to the right in the presence of increased H^+ concentration is called the *Bohr effect*.

High concentrations of 2,3-DPG are present in red cells. Levels of 2,3-DPG are increased in hypoxia, allowing greater oxygen release in the tissues. In blood stored in acid–citrate–dextrose, red cell 2,3-DPG levels decline and the haemoglobin therefore has an abnormally high affinity for oxygen, leading to poor unloading in the tissues. 2,3-DPG binds HbF less effectively than it binds HbA, facilitating transplacental oxygen transfer.

The globin genes

The genes encoding the ε-, γ-, δ-, and β-chains are found on chromosome 11. The ζ- and α-chain genes are found on chromosome 16. The α gene is duplicated so that there are two active α-chain genes on each chromosome. The genes are arranged in the order in which they are expressed during development (Fig. 5.11).

Each globin gene has three exons separated by two introns. All regions are initially transcribed. The introns are then excised from the mRNA transcript. This mature mRNA passes into the cytoplasm and binds to ribosomes. The different globin chains are synthesized separately and then come together to form a functional Hb molecule.

Incorrect excision of introns from mRNA is the most common cause of β-thalassaemia. Other causes are mutations of the regulatory sequences, mutations affecting capping and polyadenylation of mRNA, and mutations of the β-chain gene. The disorder α-thalassaemia is most commonly caused by deletion of the α gene(s). Sickle cell anaemia is caused by a single base-pair substitution in the β-chain gene.

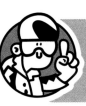

The physiological properties of haemoglobin is a very common topic in all types of exam questions. Be able to sketch Fig. 5.10 and know about the factors that affect the position of the curve.

Fig. 5.11 The globin genes.

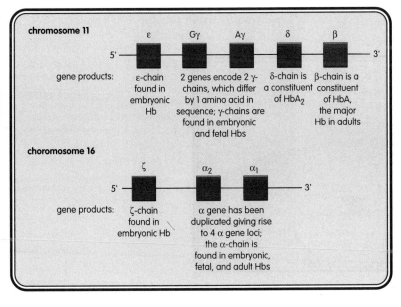

- How does the structure of haemoglobin relate to its functions?
- List the different types of haemoglobin present at different stages of development.
- What are the globin gene defects underlying the thalassaemia syndromes and sickle cell disease?
- Explain why the oxygen dissociation curve is sigmoidal and list the factors that affect its position.

THE RED CELL CYTOSKELETON

Structure

The cytoskeleton is a dense, fibrillar, protein shell that underlies the plasma membrane. The proteins of the plasma membrane, both integral and peripheral, are important constituents of the cytoskeleton (Fig. 5.12). Their band numbers refer to their mobility on electrophoresis.

Integral proteins

Integral proteins penetrate the lipid bilayer and are closely associated with it.

Band 3 protein

Band 3 protein is a glycoprotein homodimer. Its primary function is transport of anions (Cl^-, HCO_3^-). On its cytoplasmic domain, there are binding sites for ankyrin and band 4.1 protein. It also has binding sites for haemoglobin and glycolytic enzymes. The carbohydrate moiety expresses Ii blood group antigens.

Glycophorins

Glycophorins A, B, C, and D are a group of glycoproteins with the same gross structure. Each has three domains:

- Receptor.
- Transmembranous.
- Cytoplasmic.

The cytoplasmic domain of glycophorin A binds cytoskeletal proteins. The receptor domain of glycophorin A has receptors for lectins and influenza virus. The carbohydrate moiety of glycophorin A expresses MN

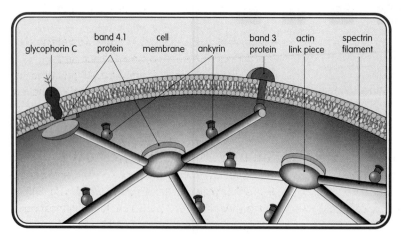

Fig. 5.12 Structure of the red cell cytoskeleton. A filamentous skeleton of the protein spectrin is anchored to the cell membrane by three main proteins (band 3 protein, ankyrin, and band 4.1 protein), with short actin pieces linking spectrin to the band 4 protein.

In the figure, labels read: glycophorin C, band 4.1 protein, cell membrane, ankyrin, band 3 protein, actin link piece, spectrin filament.

blood group antigens, and that of glycophorin B expresses N, Ss, and U blood group antigens.

Peripheral proteins
Peripheral proteins are loosely attached to the lipid bilayer.

Spectrin (bands 1 and 2)
Spectrin is the primary structural component of the cytoskeleton. The α and β subunits of spectrin twist around each other to form heterodimers, which associate to produce tetramers. Tetramers of spectrin are bound together by interactions with band 4.1 protein and actin, to form a hexagonal lattice.

Ankyrin
Ankyrin consists of bands 2.1–2.3 and 2.6. It has binding sites for the β-chain of spectrin and band 3 protein.

Band 4.1 protein
Band 4.1 protein binds spectrin, strengthening the lattice structure. It also binds band 3 protein and glycophorin.

Actin
Actin—also known as band 5—is present in the F actin configuration (short filaments formed by the assembly of G actin). It binds α- and β-spectrin, supporting the lattice of spectrin tetramers.

Function
The functions of the red cell cytoskeleton are as follows:
- It maintains cell shape and confers strength to the erythrocyte membrane, allowing the cell to withstand the stresses of the circulation.
- It permits flexibility, which is important in erythrocyte circulation.

Hereditary spherocytosis
This is an autosomal dominant disorder characterized by accelerated red cell destruction caused by deficiency or dysfunction of one of the skeletal proteins of the erythrocyte membrane. The protein most commonly implicated is spectrin (Fig. 5.13).

METABOLISM OF RED CELLS

Glucose is the principal energy source for red cells. It is taken up by facilitated diffusion via an insulin-independent pathway and is metabolized via:
- The glycolytic pathway (Embden–Meyerhoff pathway).
- The hexose monophosphate shunt.

Red cells have no mitochondria and cannot therefore aerobically metabolize glucose.

The Embden–Meyerhoff pathway
This is the glycolytic pathway common to all cells of the human body whereby glucose is metabolized to lactate (Fig. 5.14). There is a net yield of two ATP molecules, but no net NADH production.

$$\text{glucose} + 2P_i + 2ADP \rightarrow 2\ \text{lactate} + 2ATP + 2H_2O$$

Defects of glycolytic enzymes are rare. Approximately 95% are associated with pyruvate kinase and are restricted to red blood cells. Because ATP production is insufficient to maintain the structural integrity of the red cell, this leads to premature cell death, which results in a haemolytic anaemia.

The Luebering–Rapoport shunt
This—a branch of the glycolytic pathway—generates 2,3-diphosphoglycerate (2,3-DPG) as illustrated in Fig. 5.15.

Trace amounts of 2,3-DPG are found in most cells, but high concentrations are found in red cells, where

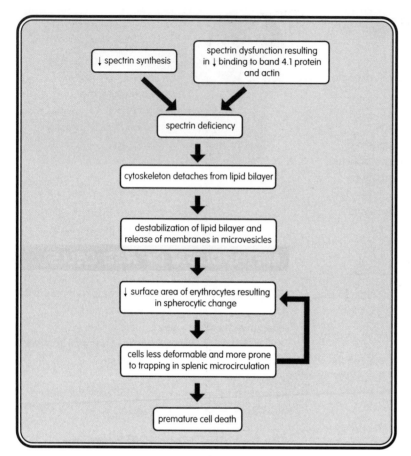

Fig. 5.13 Mechanism of spherocytosis and premature cell death in hereditary spherocytosis due to spectrin deficiency.

it is important in regulating the affinity of haemoglobin for oxygen. Between 15 and 25% of glucose passing through the glycolytic pathway enters this shunt. In doing so, the reaction catalysed by phosphoglycerate kinase is bypassed, and therefore no net ATP is produced.

The hexose monophosphate shunt

This is also known as the pentose phosphate pathway. Under normal conditions, 5% of the glucose metabolized by the red cell passes through an oxidative pathway of metabolism, the hexose monophosphate (HMP) shunt (Fig. 5.16). There is no net ATP yield, but two NADPH molecules are produced per molecule of glucose-6-phosphate

entering the shunt. The major proportion of the cell's NADPH is produced in this way.

The first three reactions constitute the irreversible oxidative portion of the pathway and are the sites of NADPH production. The remainder of the pathway is non-oxidative and, in addition to glycolytic intermediates, produces ribose-5-phosphate, which is used for nucleotide synthesis. NADPH is important in erythrocytes because it reduces oxidized glutathione (GSSG). Reduced glutathione (GSH) is required for the detoxification of oxidants.

Glucose-6-phosphate dehydrogenase deficiency is an X-linked disorder characterized by a lack of the enzyme or by a dysfunctional enzyme. Patients are usually asymptomatic, but oxidant stress can induce acute episodes of haemolysis (Fig. 5.17).

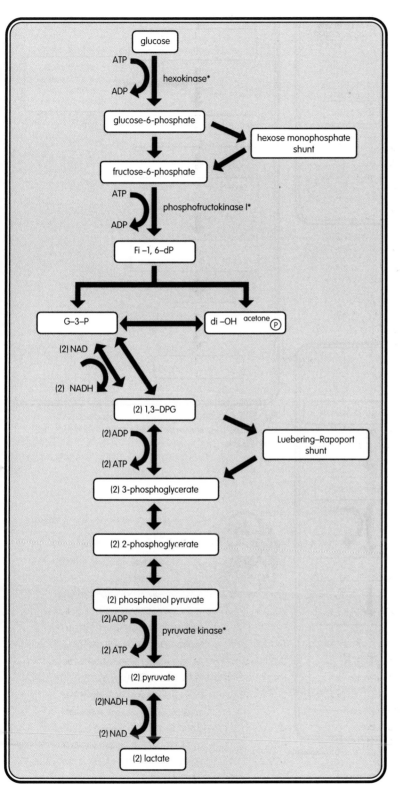

Fig. 5.14 The Embden–Meyerhoff pathway. *These enzymes catalyse the three rate-limiting steps of glycolysis.

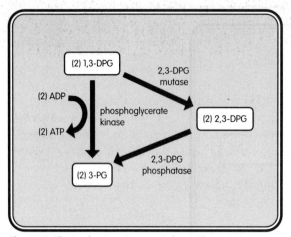

Fig. 5.15 The Luebering–Rapoport shunt. The reaction shown is per molecule of glucose. (DPG, diphosphoglycerate.)

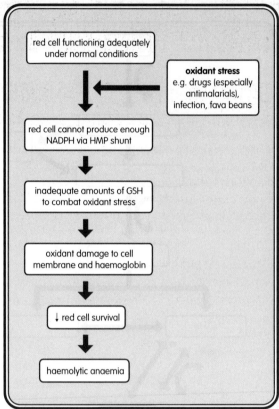

Fig. 5.17 Mechanism of haemolysis in glucose-6-phosphate dehydrogenase deficiency. (GSH, reduced glutathione.)

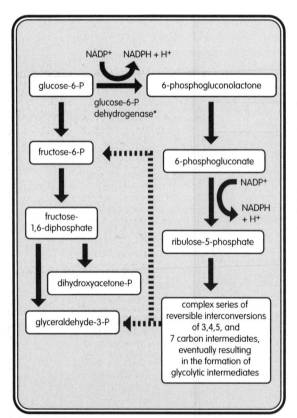

Fig. 5.16 The hexose monophosphate shunt. This simplified representation shows the oxidative portion of the cycle. *Glucose-6-phosphate dehydrogenase catalyses the rate-limiting step of the pathway.

- ○ **Summarize the pathways by which glucose is metabolized by the red cell.**
- ○ **What is the role of the Luebering–Rapoport shunt in 2,3-DPG production?**
- ○ **What is the role of the hexose monophosphate shunt in the maintenance of red cell integrity?**
- ○ **List the consequences of defects of these pathways.**

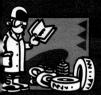

6. Haemostasis

PLATELETS AND BLOOD COAGULATION

Platelets are derived from megakaryocyte cytoplasm in the bone marrow. Their normal lifespan is 7–10 days and their mean diameter is 2–3 μm. The normal concentration of platelets in blood is $150–400 \times 10^9$/L. Up to a third of platelets are sequestered in the spleen at any one time.

Platelet structure

Platelets are non-nucleated, disc-shaped, granule-containing cells (Fig. 6.1). They contain a surface-connected canalicular system through which granule contents may be released. A circumferential microtubular band maintains the normal circulating discoid shape. Platelet endoplasmic reticulum forms a dense tubular system. It may be the site of prostaglandin and thromboxane A_2 (TxA_2) production.

Platelet production

Megakaryocytes are produced from a haemopoietic stem cell (Fig. 6.2).

Megakaryocytes mature by endomitosis, whereby cytoplasmic volume expands as the

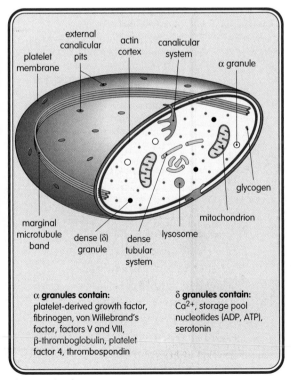

α granules contain:
platelet-derived growth factor, fibrinogen, von Willebrand's factor, factors V and VIII, β-thromboglobulin, platelet factor 4, thrombospondin

δ granules contain:
Ca^{2+}, storage pool nucleotides (ADP, ATP), serotonin

Fig. 6.1 Platelet structure.

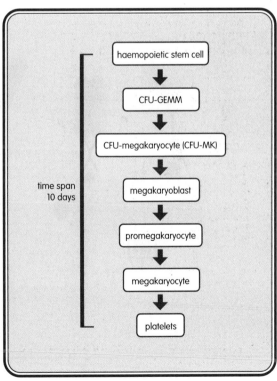

Fig. 6.2 Platelet production.

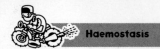

number of nuclear lobes increase. The megakaryocyte is polyploid, resulting from nuclear replication without mitosis. Each megakaryocyte can produce 2000–7000 platelets. Platelet production is governed by:

- Negative feedback control based on the number of circulating platelets.
- Thrombopoietin release (leads to an increase in platelet numbers).
- Interleukin-3 (IL-3) and granulocyte–macrophage colony stimulating factor (GM-CSF)—these stimulate CFU-megakaryocyte (CFU-MK).

Platelet function

Platelet plasma membranes contain glycoproteins, which are essential in mediating platelet–platelet and subendothelial connective tissue–platelet interaction (Fig. 6.3).

Examples of glycoprotein (GP) binding are as follows:
- GPIa binds collagen.
- GPIb and GPIIb/IIIa bind von Willebrand's factor (vWF). vWF has two binding sites, one for exposed microfibrils and another for GPIb. It is synthesized by endothelial cells and megakaryocytes.
- GPIIb/IIIa also binds fibrinogen.

Release reaction

Within 1–2 seconds of adhesion, platelets change from discs to spheres with numerous cytoplasmic projections, promoting platelet–platelet interactions. Degranulation and release of granule contents occurs.

Platelet aggregation

Released contents of α granules and dense granules promote further platelet adhesion and aggregation; for example, ADP released from

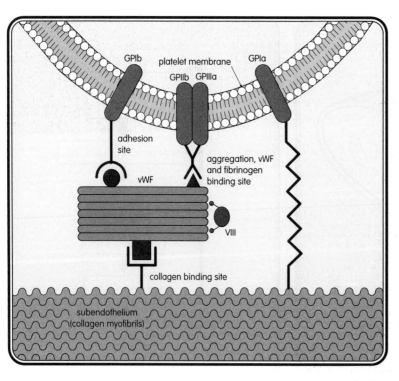

Fig. 6.3 Platelet adhesion. Damage to the vessel wall exposes subendothelial microfibrils which bind von Willebrand's factor (vWF). This in turn interacts with platelets via GPIb (calcium required) and leads to GPIIb/IIa receptor exposure. This receptor acts as a secondary binding site for vWF. Platelet binding to collagen types I, II, and III on the subendothelium occurs via GPIa and adhesion is complete.

dense granules alters the surface configuration of platelets circulating locally in the blood, promoting aggregation. Subendothelial collagen and thrombin potentiate platelet adhesion and aggregation by promoting ADP release and TxA_2 production.

Platelet aggregation leads to the exposure of GPIIb/IIIa, which binds plasma fibrinogen and promotes aggregation onto platelets already bound to the subendothelium, vWF, and collagen. A self-propagating system is set in motion which promotes further platelet adhesion and aggregation and causes further release of ADP and TxA_2. This results in the formation of a platelet plug. Aggregation is made irreversible by:

- High levels of ADP.
- Platelet release products.
- Platelet contractile proteins.

Thrombin encourages platelet adhesion by converting fibrinogen to fibrin and strengthening the platelet plug. Prostacyclin (PGI_2), released by the endothelial cell membrane, inhibits platelet aggregation and inhibits platelet interaction with normal endothelium (Fig. 6.4).

Procoagulant function
Platelet aggregation leads to the rearrangement of membrane phospholipid (platelet factor III), providing an ideal site for important procoagulant reactions to take place. These result in the formation of factor Xa (see p. 80).

Tissue repair
The α granules of platelets contain platelet-derived growth factor (PDGF), which is mitogenic for vascular smooth muscle cells and fibroblasts and stimulates wound healing.

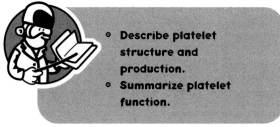

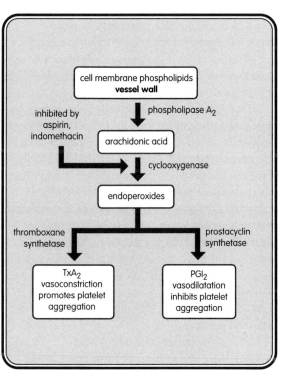

Fig. 6.4 Pathway of thromboxane A_2 (TxA_2) and prostacyclin (PGI_2) production.

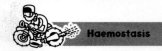

THE COAGULATION CASCADE

The coagulation cascade involves the interaction of procoagulant plasma proteins in a specific sequence. The result is the generation of thrombin, which converts soluble fibrinogen into insoluble fibrin. Fibrin strengthens and consolidates the platelet plug. The components of the coagulation cascade (Fig. 6.5) are synthesized by the liver. Endothelial cells and megakaryocytes produce vWF.

A Roman numeral followed by the suffix 'a' is used to denote the activated form of a procoagulant protein, e.g. the activated form of factor II is IIa.

With the exception of fibrinogen, coagulation factors are either one of two types:

- Proenzymes—these are transformed into active enzymes after hydrolysis of one or more peptide bonds. Examples include factors II, VII, and IX–XIII, and prekallikrein. They are all serine proteases except for factor XIII, which is a transglutaminase.

The coagulation proteins	
Factor number	**Name**
I	fibrinogen
II	prothrombin
III	tissue factor (thromboplastin)
V	labile factor
VII	proconvertin
VIII	anti-haemophilic factor
IX	Christmas factor
X	Stuart-Prower factor
XI	plasma thromboplastin antecedent
XII	Hageman factor
XIII	fibrin-stabilizing factor
	prekallikrein
	high-molecular-weight kininogen (HMWK)

Fig. 6.5 Components of the coagulation cascade.

- Co-factors—these are not converted into active enzymes, but aid and accelerate other enzymatic reactions. Examples include factors III, V, and VIII, and high-molecular-weight kininogen (HMWK).

The coagulation cascade is an amplification pathway—consequently, for example, one molecule of activated factor XI (XIa) may eventually generate up to 2×10^8 molecules of fibrin.

Blood coagulation

Two interdependent coagulation pathways are recognized:

- The intrinsic pathway.
- The extrinsic pathway.

The intrinsic pathway

All the necessary components for the intrinsic pathway are present in plasma. It is activated by exposure of blood to negatively charged surfaces such as subendothelial collagen and microfibrils, basement membrane, and lipopolysaccharide (Fig. 6.6). A conformational change in factor XII results in the conversion of prekallikrein to kallikrein. Kallikrein fully activates factor XII in a process known as reciprocal proteolytic activation. Factor XIIa catalyses conversion of factor XI to factor XIa. HMWK acts as a cofactor for all these reactions by binding factor XI and prekallikrein to the activating surface.

Factor XIa then activates factor IX. The platelet membrane phospholipid (platelet factor III) provides the template on which factor IXa activates factor X (factor VIII acts as a cofactor). Factor Xa then activates factor II (prothrombin; factor V acts as a cofactor). Calcium ions are required for both of these steps. Prothrombin is converted to thrombin. The latter cleaves fibrinogen into fibrin monomers, which form an unstable polymer. Factor XIII (fibrin-stabilizing factor) is activated by thrombin and calcium ions, and acts to consolidate the fibrin clot by catalysing the formation of covalent bonds between adjacent fibrin molecules.

The intrinsic pathway may also be activated by two other mechanisms:

- Factor XI can be activated by thrombin.
- Factor VIIa of the extrinsic pathway may convert factor IX to its active form.

The extrinsic pathway

Tissue factor (TF; factor III) released from damaged tissue complexes with plasma factor VII in the presence of calcium ions. Factor VII binds via its γ-carboxyglutamic acid residues and is converted to its active form (see Fig. 6.6). The TF–VIIa complex then activates factor X. A common final pathway for the intrinsic and extrinsic systems is reached at this point. The pro-cofactors V and VIII are activated by thrombin (positive feedback) and at the same time protein C may be activated to limit coagulation (negative feedback).

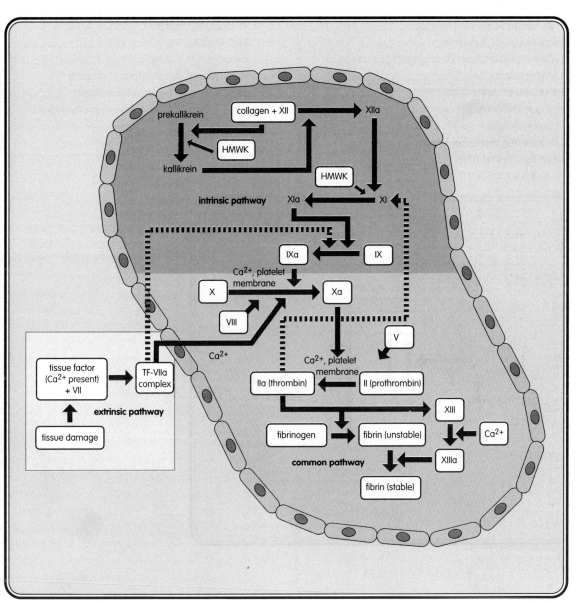

Fig. 6.6 Intrinsic and extrinsic pathways of blood coagulation.

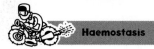
Role of vitamin K and calcium ions in coagulation

Factors II, VII, IX, and X and proteins C and S are dependent on vitamin K for post-translational modification (Fig. 6.7). Vitamin K acts as a cofactor for the γ-carboxylation of glutamic acid residues, enabling these molecules to bind calcium and form complexes with the platelet phospholipid membrane. In the absence of vitamin K, factors II, VII, IX, and X:

- Do not undergo γ-carboxylation.
- Cannot bind calcium ions
- Are unable to attach onto platelet phospholipid membranes.
- Are known as proteins induced by vitamin K absence (PIVKA).

Consequently, negligible levels of prothrombin are converted into thrombin.

Blood storage

Adequate levels of calcium ions are essential for clotting. Blood can be stored by reducing calcium ion levels below the clotting threshold. This is done in two ways:

- By using citrate ions, which deionize the calcium.
- By precipitating calcium with ions such as oxalate.

Warfarin

Warfarin is a vitamin K antagonist. It inhibits the γ-carboxylation of the vitamin-K-dependent factors II, VII, IX, and X and proteins C and S (see Fig. 6.7). After the first dose, the activity of the factors declines in the circulation in the order VII, IX, X, and II, dependent on half-life. Warfarin therapy is controlled by measuring the International Normalized Ratio (INR)—the ratio of prothrombin time to control prothrombin time.

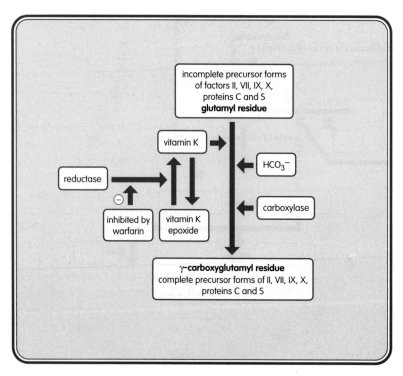

Fig. 6.7 Post-translational modification of the vitamin-K-dependent factors. The glutamyl residue of the coagulation factors undergoes γ-carboxylation and can then bind calcium ions and attach onto platelet phospholipid membranes.

Regulatory pathways of coagulation

Because of anticoagulant mechanisms present in the plasma, coagulation is normally restricted to the site of injury.

Proteins C and S

These are vitamin-K-dependent inhibitors of coagulation. Protein C, a serine protease, becomes activated by the thrombin–thrombomodulin complex on the endothelial surface. Activated protein C destroys factors Va and VIIIa, thereby inhibiting the conversion of prothrombin to thrombin by factor Xa. Protein S potentiates the activity of protein C. Activated protein C also augments fibrinolysis.

Antithrombin III and heparin

Antithrombin III (ATIII) is a potent inhibitor of thrombin, but also inactivates factors IXa, Xa, and XIIa. The binding of heparin to ATIII markedly enhances its rate of enzyme degradation. This is the basis for the anticoagulant action of heparin. Low-molecular-weight heparin inhibits factor Xa more effectively than it does thrombin. As heparin does not cross the placenta, it can be used in pregnancy. Heparin therapy is monitored using the activated partial thromboplastin time (APTT)—the therapeutic range is 1.5–2.5 times the normal value.

Warfarin and heparin affect different parts of the coagulation cascade and differ in their rate of onset. These two facts determine their varying uses in clinical practice.

Clotting defects

Four basic tests are used to diagnose clotting defects:

- Prothrombin time—this estimates the activity of the extrinsic and common pathways (normal time: 10–14 seconds).
- Activated partial thromboplastin time (APTT)—this measures the activity of the intrinsic and common pathways (normal time: 30–40 seconds).
- Thrombin time—this is used when: (i) there is deficiency of fibrinogen (inherited or acquired); (ii) abnormal fibrinogen molecules are present (inherited or acquired); (iii) there is inhibition of thrombin (normal time: 14–16 seconds).
- Bleeding time—this is a measure of platelet function and of vWF. The normal time (3–8 minutes) is increased when the platelet concentration is $<75 \times 10^9$/L and in platelet dysfunction.

Fibrinolysis

Fibrin production is counterbalanced by fibrinolysis. This is part of the normal response to tissue injury. Fibrinolysis is the dissolution of fibrin into fibrin degradation products (FDPs). The serine protease plasmin is responsible for this process (Fig. 6.8). The precursor molecule plasminogen is synthesized in the liver. It is converted to plasmin by two routes:

- Intrinsic activators—derived from blood vessels or generated during blood coagulation.
- Extrinsic activators—derived from tissues.

Intrinsic activation of fibrinolysis is mediated by factors XIIa and IXa, kallikrein, and HMWK. Extrinsic activation involves the release of tissue plasminogen activator (tPA) from endothelial cells and is the most important activator of the fibrinolytic system. It is a serine protease with a strong affinity for fibrin. The fibrin–tPA complex is a more potent activator of plasminogen than tPA is alone. Fibrin increases the affinity of tPA for plasminogen and thereby confines its action to the clot. A variety of stimuli induce tPA release, including trauma, prolonged exercise, venous occlusion, stress, and thrombin.

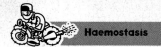
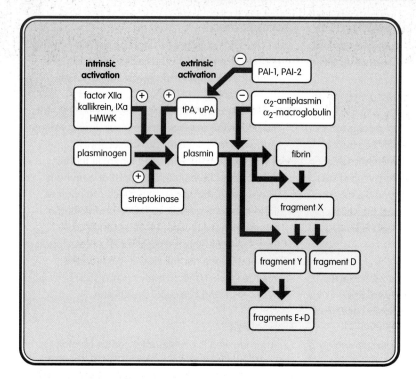

Fig. 6.8 The fibrinolytic pathway. (PAI-1 and PAI-2, plasminogen activator inhibitors 1 and 2; tPA, tissue plasminogen activator; uPA, urokinase plasminogen activator.)

Urokinase plasminogen activator (uPA), synthesized in the kidney, also activates plasminogen. Non-physiological activators of plasminogen include streptokinase (produced by haemolytic streptococci), which is increasingly used clinically as a thrombolytic agent. Plasmin has the ability to degrade fibrinogen and factors V and VIII.

The major inhibitors of circulating plasmin are α_2-antiplasmin and α_2-macroglobulin. Plasminogen activator inhibitor 1 (PAI-1) is a major inhibitor of tPA and uPA, whereas PAI-2 mainly inhibits u-PA (see Fig. 6.8). The fibrinolytic system is, therefore, controlled by specific inhibitors in an analagous manner to the coagulation system.

The fibrin–tPA complex converts plasminogen to plasmin, which then digests the fibrin onto which it is absorbed. Fibrin degradation gives rise to split products, the so-called fibrin degradation products (FDPs). Initial cleavage gives rise to fragment X, which undergoes further proteolysis to produce fragments Y and D. Fragment X acts as a competitive inhibitor of thrombin by binding it via specific sites. Fragment Y acts as a competitive inhibitor of fibrin polymerization.

Further cleavage of fragment Y produces fragment E and a second fragment D.

- Describe the intrinsic and extrinsic coagulation pathways.
- What is the role of vitamin K and calcium in coagulation?
- Describe the mode of action of warfarin.
- Summarize the regulatory pathways of coagulation.
- Describe the fibrinolytic pathway and the inhibitors of fibrinolysis.

7. Serum Proteins

NORMAL SERUM PROTEINS

The following definitions are important here:
- Serum—this is plasma minus components that contribute towards the formation of a fibrin clot.
- Paraprotein—this is a monoclonal immunoglobulin found in the serum, characteristically in multiple myeloma or Waldenstrom's macroglobulinaemia.

Serum is used in preference to plasma for electrophoretic assessment because the fibrinogen found in plasma produces a band in the β_1 region which could be mistaken for a paraprotein. When electrophoresis is carried out on cellulose acetate or agarose gel, the pattern shown in Fig. 7.1 is obtained.

Albumin

Albumin is the most abundant serum protein and is the main protein synthesized by the liver. It is the principal agent in maintaining the oncotic pressure (osmotic pressure due to proteins) of plasma. In addition, it acts as a transport protein for calcium, thyroid hormones, and fatty acids, and also binds unconjugated bilirubin.

Alpha-1-globulins
Alpha-1-antitrypsin

Alpha-1-antitrypsin (α_1-AT) is a glycoprotein synthesized by the liver and secreted into the bloodstream. It accounts for 90% of the α_1-globulin band. It is a protease inhibitor (PI) with three genetic variants, classified on the basis of their electrophoretic mobility:
- M (medium).
- S (slow).
- Z (very slow).

The most common allele is PiM. Heterozygous states are not significant as PiMZ heterozygotes produce 60% of normal circulating levels of α_1-AT and have only a slightly increased risk of lung disease such as emphysema.

Homozygotes for the PiZ allele (PiZZ) possess only 15% of normal circulating α_1-AT levels. This is because the α_1-AT produced by this phenotype cannot be

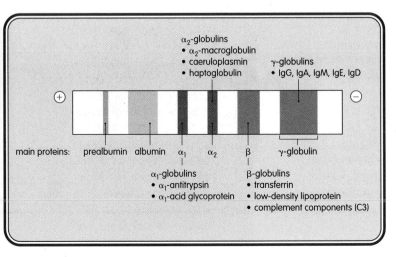

Fig. 7.1 Normal pattern of serum proteins on serum electrophoresis.

readily secreted from the liver, where it accumulates and causes liver damage. It is associated with neonatal hepatitis, and childhood and adult cirrhosis. Rarely, hepatocellular carcinoma also occurs. In addition, the α_1-AT is unable to diffuse into the lungs and consequently the actions of neutrophil elastase go unchecked. A deficiency of α_1-AT, therefore, is associated with panacinar emphysema. Alpha-1 antitrypsin is also an acute phase protein which is raised in acute inflammatory states; however, the level only rises to half the normal in PiZZ homozygotes during an acute phase response.

Alpha-1 antitrypsin deficiency can cause hepatitis and pulmonary disease.

Alpha-2-globulins
Haptoglobulin
The main function of haptoglobulin (HP) is to bind haemoglobin (Hb) released from lysed red blood cells. The HP–Hb complex is cleared by the reticuloendothelial system and the rate of removal increases if the rate of Hb release increases. A low HP concentration can therefore be indicative of an increased rate of haemolysis. HP is also an acute phase protein.

Alpha-2-macroglobulin
Alpha-2-macroglobulin is a protease inhibitor like α_1-AT, but has a broader range of activity.

Caeruloplasmin
Caeruloplasmin is a carrier protein for copper, as well as being an acute phase protein. It is deficient in Wilson's disease.

Beta-globulins
Transferrin
Transferrin is the major transport protein for iron in the plasma. Plasma transferrin is typically 30% saturated with iron; this figure rises to 100% in haemochromatosis.

Low-density lipoprotein
Low-density lipoprotein (LDL) is the major carrier of cholesterol in the form of cholesteryl ester.

Complement components
Details of complement components can be found in Chapter 3.

Gamma-globulins
The γ-globulins comprise the immunoglobulins and are discussed in Chapter 3.

The clinical significance of abnormalities of these proteins on serum electrophoresis is detailed in Fig. 7.2.

Serum proteins—electrophoresis and clinical significance of abnormalities	
Electrophoretic pattern	**Diagnostic inference**
decrease in albumin, α_1-globulin, and γ-globulins; increase in α_2-globulin and β-globulin	nephrotic syndrome
decrease in albumin; diffuse increase in γ-globulins, resulting in $\beta\gamma$ fusion	cirrhosis
decrease in α_1-globulin band	α_1-AT deficiency
decrease in γ-globulin band	hypogammaglobulinaemia
increase in γ-globulin band	diffuse hypergammaglobulinaemia
distinct band in γ-globulin region	paraprotein

Fig. 7.2 Clinical significance of abnormalities of plasma proteins on serum electrophoresis.

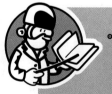

- **Sketch the normal band pattern obtained on serum electrophoresis.**
- **List the functions of the various serum proteins.**
- **What is the clinical significance of abnormalities found on serum electrophoresis?**

ACUTE PHASE PROTEINS

The acute phase response is the systemic reaction to infection or tissue injury. Stimuli that induce the acute phase include:

- Inflammation.
- Infections.
- Tissue necrosis, e.g. myocardial infarction.
- Malignancy.
- Chemicals.
- Trauma.

The acute phase response is characterized by an alteration in the concentration of a number of plasma proteins—the so-called acute phase proteins. These include:

- C-reactive protein.
- Serum amyloid A.
- Complement components.
- Fibrinogen.
- Alpha-1 antitrypsin.
- Caeruloplasmin.
- Haptoglobulin.

This change in plasma concentration is accompanied by fever, leucocytosis, thrombocytosis, and catabolism of muscle proteins. Synthesis of acute phase proteins (APPs) by the liver is enhanced by cytokines secreted by macrophages and endothelial cells. The two main APPs are C-reactive protein (CRP) and serum amyloid A (SAA)

The extent of the rise in the plasma concentration of different APPs varies:

- Increase of 50% above normal levels— caeruloplasmin.
- Increase of several fold above normal levels—α_1-glycoprotein, α_1-proteinase inhibitor, haptoglobulin, fibrinogen.
- Increase of 100–1000 fold—CRP, SAA.

In contrast, the concentration of other plasma proteins, most notably albumin and transferrin, falls.

C-reactive protein

The exact function of CRP in the acute phase response is unknown. Levels of CRP rise within hours of tissue injury or infection. CRP can activate the classical complement pathway and can bind to and modulate the behaviour of phagocytic cells. CRP elevation can be slight (e.g. cerebrovascular accident), moderate (e.g. myocardial infarction), or marked (e.g. bacterial infections).

Serum amyloid A

The function of SAA is unclear, but its levels rise within hours of tissue injury or infection. It may function as an opsonin. Inflammatory disorders in which SAA levels are raised include inflammatory bowel disease and rheumatoid arthritis. Persistent elevation of SAA may lead to its deposition in tissues.

Other acute phase proteins

Plasma levels of other APPs are not routinely measured because they rise relatively slowly following injury or infection and the extent of the increase is relatively small in comparison to that of CRP or SAA.

Erythrocyte sedimentation rate

The erythrocyte sedimentation rate (ESR) is an index of the acute phase response. It is especially representative of the concentration of fibrinogen and α-globulins. Elevated fibrinogen levels cause red cells to form stacks (rouleaux), which sediment more rapidly than individual blood cells. The ESR has been used as a standard test for the acute phase response although CRP levels are increasingly being used.

- Describe the nature of the acute phase response.
- How do the levels of individual acute phase proteins vary in infection or tissue injury?
- What is the relevance of acute phase proteins to clinical tests?

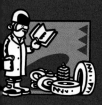

8. Serology and Blood Transfusion

RED CELL ANTIGENS

ABO antigens

Human red cells have a variety of antigens on their surface. The ABO system was the first to be discovered and remains the most important. Each ABO antigen consists of a chain of sugars attached to a lipid or protein in the red cell membrane. ABO antigen status is inherited and consists of three allelic genes: A, B, and O. The A and B genes both code for enzymes known as transferases. These convert a basic antigen, H (coded for by the H gene and inherited as HH or Hh), found on every red cell membrane, into either A or B antigens. The O gene is amorphous, i.e. it has no effect on antigenic structure and leaves antigen H unchanged. Six different genotypes can give rise to four possible phenotypes (Fig. 8.1).

Within the first 6 months of life, individuals generate IgM antibodies against those blood group antigens (either A or B or both) that are not present on their own cells. This occurs because of exposure to naturally occurring A-like and B-like antigens found in intestinal bacteria and food substances. These antibodies facilitate agglutination and subsequent haemolysis of red blood cells *in vivo*. Therefore, transfusion of blood of group A into a group O recipient will result in destruction of the donor red cells owing to the presence of anti-A antibodies in the recipient's serum. It is thus important that the transfused blood is ABO-compatible with the recipient's blood.

Ideally, ABO-identical donors are selected. When this is not possible, compatible blood donors are chosen. Blood cells of group O are not affected by anti-A and anti-B antibodies and can therefore be given to patients of any blood group. Consequently, blood group O is referred to as the universal donor. Conversely, AB individuals do not possess anti-A or anti-B antibodies and can receive any blood group. They are universal recipients.

Rhesus antigens

Rhesus (Rh) antigens are good immunogens and the antibodies generated are clinically important. The system consists of two closely linked genes, present on chromosome 1, which are inherited *en bloc*:

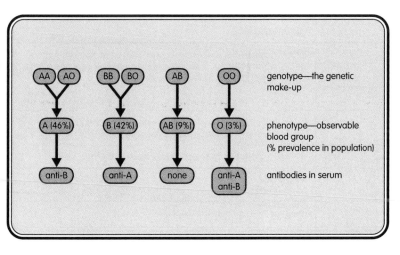

Fig. 8.1 Genotypes and phenotypes of ABO blood groups.

- RhCE—encoding C, c, E, and e antigens.
- RhD—encoding the D antigen.

Absence of the D antigen is denoted 'd'. The most important antigen is the D antigen because it is the strongest immunogen. By convention, individuals possessing this antigen are termed Rhesus positive (Rh +ve) and those lacking the D antigen are Rhesus negative (Rh −ve). Rh +ve individuals are DD (homozygous) or Dd (heterozygous), and Rh −ve individuals are dd. Approximately 85% of Caucasians are Rh +ve and 15% are Rh −ve.

Unlike the naturally occurring antibodies of the ABO system, anti-D antibodies are generated only after a Rh −ve individual is exposed to Rh +ve red cells. All antibodies produced are IgG. Approximately 70% of Rh −ve individuals have titres of anti-D antibodies after receiving Rh +ve blood and they may develop transfusion reactions when re-transfused with Rh +ve blood.

RhD haemolytic disease of the newborn

If a Rh −ve mother is carrying a Rh +ve fetus, there is a risk of sensitization. This usually occurs at birth, when small amounts of Rh +ve fetal blood leak into the Rh −ve maternal circulation. Subsequently, mothers develop titres of IgG antibodies which are capable of crossing the placenta and entering the fetal circulation during the course of the second pregnancy. If the second fetus is Rh +ve, the IgG antibodies can bind to the fetal red cells, inducing haemolysis. In its most severe form, this results in hydrops fetalis.

Prevention of RhD haemolytic disease of the newborn
If anti-D IgG is administered intramuscularly to the Rh −ve mother at 28 weeks and within 72 hours of the birth, the D antigen on fetal red blood cells in the maternal circulation becomes coated with it, preventing a maternal immune response. The Rh +ve red blood cell–anti-D antibody complex is then removed in the maternal reticuloendothelial system (RES). The dose of anti-D IgG can be adjusted depending on the volume of fetal red blood cells in the maternal circulation, as estimated by the Kleihauer technique. Anti-D antibody is also used following abortion in Rh −ve women and following transfusion of Rh +ve blood into Rh −ve individuals.

Other red cell antigens
Other red cell antigens are listed in Fig. 8.2.

Other red cell antigens		
Blood group system	**Common alleles**	**Clinical significance**
Kell	K, k	antigen-negative individuals produce antibodies against antigen-positive RBCs due to sensitization during either transfusion or pregnancy, resulting in haemolysis and HDN; especially true for K antigen
Duffy	Fy^a, Fy^b	
Kidd	Jk^a, Jk^b	
I-i	I, i	found on almost all human RBCs; anti-I antibodies are IgM subtype and found in cold autoimmune haemolytic anaemia
MNSs	M, N, S, s	only anti-S antibodies cause clinically significant haemolysis
P system	P	the IgG autoantibody (Donath–Landsteiner) directed against P antigen is found in patients with paroxysmal cold haemoglobinuria
Lewis antigen	Le^a, Le^b	usually of no clinical significance

Fig. 8.2 Other red cell antigens (HDN, haemolytic disease of the newborn.

In Rhesus disease, the first child is almost always unaffected. However, subsequent pregnancies are at risk.

Prevention of RhD haemolytic disease of the newborn is a very common exam topic and should be understood well.

- ○ **Describe the ABO and Rhesus blood group systems.**
- ○ **List the other red cell antigens and the possible clinical problems associated with them.**
- ○ **What is haemolytic disease of the newborn?**

BLOOD TRANSFUSION

The transfusion reaction

Transfusion of incompatible blood results in transfusion reactions, the most severe—as well as the most preventable—being acute haemolytic transfusion reactions.

Acute haemolytic transfusion reactions

Acute haemolytic transfusion reactions are caused by the destruction of donor red blood cells by antibodies (IgG or IgM) present in the recipient's serum. Haemolysis can be intravascular as a result of complement fixation by IgM antibodies (ABO incompatibility). Activation of complement generates C3a and C5a, which cause vasodilatation, increased vascular permeability, and neutrophil chemotaxis.

Symptoms may occur within a few minutes or may take several hours to develop. They include pain, fever, flushing, urticaria, and diarrhoea and vomiting. Shock results from the profound hypotension caused by the release of vasoactive substances, and renal failure may result from renal tubular necrosis. Release of tissue thromboplastin from lysed red cells may lead to disseminated intravascular coagulation (DIC). Death occurs in

15% of cases of ABO incompatibility and usually results from severe DIC or renal failure.

Extravascular haemolysis results from incompatibilities of the Rh, Kell, Duffy, and Kidd blood group systems. Anti-blood-system antibodies produced by the recipient are unable to bind complement effectively and the antibody-coated red blood cells are removed extravascularly by the RES.

Cross-matching blood

It is important to label samples accurately before blood transfusions in order to prevent potentially fatal transfusion reactions. The procedure for obtaining compatible blood comprises three separate steps:

1. ABO and Rh blood groups of the recipient are determined.
2. An antibody screen is carried out on the recipient's blood—the recipient's serum is tested against a standard pool of red cells bearing the most important red cell antigens. The aim is to detect antibodies to blood group antigens other than those of the ABO and Rh systems.
3. Each unit of donor blood to be transfused is then tested against the patient's serum to identify atypical antibodies.

Emergency transfusions

Patients requiring emergency transfusions, e.g. for acute haemorrhage, should receive either:

- Whole blood containing red cells, fluid, electrolytes, and plasma proteins.
- Red cells suspended in SAG-M (saline-adenine-glucose-mannitol—a nutrient solution), which contains no plasma and therefore no blood group antibodies and no proteins.

Other blood products

Platelets

Platelets are stored at room temperature and have a half-life of 4–5 days. They may be obtained from a pool of 6–10 blood donors or via apheresis, when platelets from a single donor are collected by automated methods.

Fresh frozen plasma

Fresh frozen plasma (FFP) contains albumin, immunoglobulins, and all the clotting factors. Indications for FFP transfusion include:

- Multiple clotting factor deficiencies, e.g. severe liver disease, warfarin overdose, massive transfusion (more than 10 units within 24 hours).
- Specific coagulation factor replacement.
- Plasma loss, e.g. due to burns.

Compatibility is the opposite to that for red cells.

Cryoprecipitate

Cryoprecipitate is the insoluble precipitate formed when FFP is thawed at $4°C$. It contains clotting factors including factor VIII, von Willebrand's factor (vWF), factor XIII, and fibrinogen, and is given to control bleeding associated with defects thereof.

Clotting factor concentrates

Specific clotting factor concentrates can be given to patients with clotting factor deficiencies.

For example, factors VIII and IX are used for the treatment and prevention of bleeding in haemophilia A and B, respectively.

- **Describe the transfusion reaction and its possible consequences.**
- **Summarize cross-matching of blood.**
- **Which blood products should be given in an emergency blood transfusion?**
- **What are the indications for transfusion of fresh frozen plasma?**

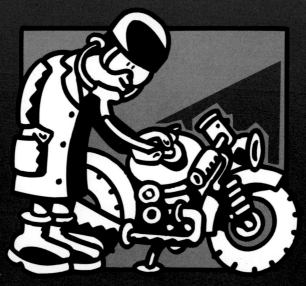

CLINICAL
ASSESSMENT

9. **Taking a History** 95

10. **Clinical Examination** 101

11. **Further Investigations** 105

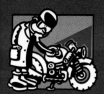

9. Taking a History

Before starting to take a history, always introduce yourself to the patient. Be polite at all times, maintain good eye contact, and try to build up a rapport with the patient.

STRUCTURE OF A HISTORY

Although the facts may be obtained in any order, the written history must be presented in a certain sequence. Keep these headings in mind whilst talking to the patient, and present the history as follows:
- Name, age, sex, and ethnic group of patient.
- Background.
- Presenting complaint.
- History of presenting complaint.
- Past medical history.
- Drug history.
- Family history.
- Social history.
- Review of systems.
- Summary.

Background

When presenting a history, put the patient's current problem into context by outlining any relevant background information before launching into the details of the presenting complaint. For example, in a patient presenting with clinical features of a pneumonia, the fact that he or she has recently had a renal transplant and is on high-dose immunosuppressive therapy is of great relevance and should be mentioned before the history of the pneumonia is described.

Presenting complaint

Present a summary of the patient's current problem, as described by him or her, of not more than one or two lines in length: for example, 'Mr X has a 6-month history of fever and weight loss.'

History of presenting complaint

This is the most important part of the history and you will probably spend most of your time on this section. Use a combination of open and closed questions. For example, a good way of starting is by asking the patient, 'Would you like to tell me about your problems?' (an open question), thus allowing them to tell you the story in their own words. If the patient mentions specific symptoms, e.g. chest pain, it is then appropriate to focus upon and ask closed questions relevant to the symptom, e.g. 'Where is the pain?', 'Does the pain spread elsewhere?'.

Although this may be difficult at first, it is vital to consider in your mind what the differential diagnoses may be whilst you are taking the history so that you can then ask specific questions relating to those diagnoses. For example, in a patient presenting with haematemesis, it is necessary ask about symptoms of peptic ulcer disease (e.g. epigastric pain, nausea, weight loss, etc.). It is useful to present these findings (both positive and negative) as you describe the symptoms.

When presenting a history, start by stating when the patient was last well and then list the symptoms in chronological order of onset. For any symptom, the following pieces of information must be obtained:
- Onset (i.e. sudden or gradual).
- Duration.
- Frequency.
- Precipitating and relieving factors.
- Associated symptoms.
- Progression since onset (i.e. 'Is it getting better or worse, or is it the same?').

For the symptom of pain, also ask about:
- Site.
- Character, e.g. stabbing or colicky.
- Radiation.

Past medical history

It is valuable to ask the patient the following questions:

- Do you have any other medical problems?
- Have you had any serious illnesses?
- Have you ever had to take excessive time off work due to illness?
- Have you been admitted to hospital before?
- Have you had any operations?

A useful battery of conditions to ask about are diabetes mellitus, asthma, epilepsy, myocardial infarction, stroke, tuberculosis, rheumatic fever, anaemia, and jaundice.

Drug history

Ask about and list the names and doses of the drugs that the patient is taking. Allergies should also be mentioned in this section.

Family history

Ask the patient about their parents, siblings, and children. If there is a family history of a relevant disorder, especially if it is a inherited condition, it is a good idea to draw a family tree.

Social history

Ask about:

- Risk habits, e.g. smoking, alcohol consumption.
- Marital status and any children.
- Finance and accommodation.
- Occupation.
- Recent travel abroad.

Review of systems

This comprises a set of routine questions that can be asked at the end of the history or after the history of the presenting complaint (Fig. 9.1).

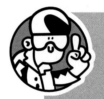

Remember to use language that the patient can understand. Beware of using terms like orthopnoea and dysphagia when questioning patients. Make sure that you are able to describe these symptoms to patients in lay terms.

Fig. 9.1 Review of systems.

System	Symptoms to ask about
Review of systems	
general	change in appetite or weight; fatigue; fever; night sweats; general wellbeing
respiratory	dyspnoea, wheeze, cough, sputum production, haemoptysis
cardiovascular	chest pain, palpitations, exercise tolerance, orthopnoea, paroxysmal nocturnal dyspnoea, ankle swelling, claudication
gastrointestinal	nausea and vomiting, dysphagia, indigestion, abdominal pain, bowel habits, rectal bleeding
urinary	loin pain, frequency, dribbling, dysuria, nocturia, haematuria, incontinence
nervous system	headaches; fits; faints; changes in vision, hearing, speech, or memory; sensory or motor changes; bladder or bowel disturbance; anxiety and depression; sleep patterns
musculoskeletal	pain, stiffness, or swelling of the joints
skin	rashes

Summary

At the end of your presentation, always summarize the history, concentrating on the positive and the important negative findings, and then try and suggest a list of differential diagnoses.

○ **Describe how you would take a history.**

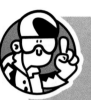

The key to successful history taking is practice. Clerk as many patients as you can and always try and present your history to someone, even if it's just another student!

COMMON PRESENTING COMPLAINTS

Anaemia

If you suspect a diagnosis of anaemia, you should ask yourself certain questions (Fig. 9.2). A diagnostic algorithm, such as the one shown in Fig. 9.3, can be used to determine the type of anaemia.

Bleeding

If you suspect a bleeding disorder, you should ask yourself certain questions (Fig. 9.4). A diagnostic algorithm, such as the one shown in Fig. 9.5, can be used to determine the type of bleeding disorder.

Questions to ask when considering differential diagnoses of anaemia	
Question	**Comment**
Is the patient's diet adequate?	an inadequate diet can be a cause of iron deficiency or megaloblastic anaemia
Are there any symptoms suggesting malabsorption, e.g. diarrhoea, weight loss?	malabsorption of iron, vitamin B_{12}, or folate can result in anaemia
Does the patient have any neurological symptoms? Does the patient have disease of the terminal ileum?	positive responses are suggestive of vitamin B_{12} deficiency
Is there a history suggestive of chronic blood loss?	e.g. menorrhagia and gastrointestinal blood loss
Is the patient jaundiced?	a positive response is suggestive of a haemolytic disorder
Is there a family history of anaemia?	a positive history is especially important in certain racial groups
Does the patient have a chronic illness?	anaemia of chronic disease
Does the patient have any features of malignancy?	anaemia can be a presenting feature of malignancy
Is the patient taking any drugs that could cause anaemia?	e.g. aspirin can cause gastrointestinal bleeding, methotrexate causes folate deficiency

Fig. 9.2 Questions to ask when considering differential diagnoses of anaemia.

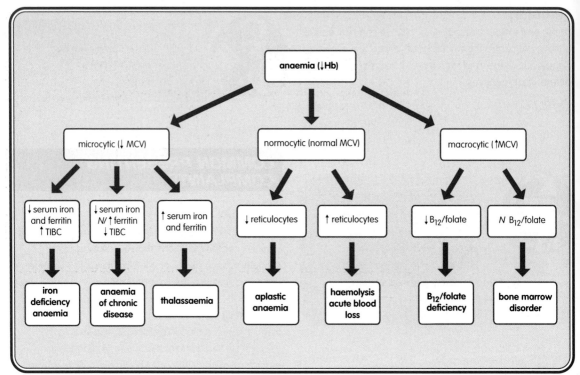

Fig. 9.3 Diagnostic algorithm for anaemia. (MCV, mean cell volume; N, normal; TIBC, total iron-binding capacity.)

Questions to ask when considering differential diagnoses of bleeding	
Question	**Comment**
What is the site of the bleed?	skin and mucous membrane bleeds suggest a platelet disorder; joint and muscle bleeds suggest a coagulation cascade disorder
Are there any factors that precipitate the bleeding or does it occur spontaneously?	spontaneous bleeds indicate a more severe disorder than bleeding secondary to trauma
Is there any excessive bleeding after surgery, e.g. tooth extraction, and if so, when does it start?	immediate bleeding suggests defective platelet function, whereas delayed bleeding suggests a defect of the coagulation cascade
How long have the symptoms of bleeding been evident?	long-standing bleeding suggests a congenital disorder
Is there a family history of a bleeding disorder?	a positive response suggests a hereditary disorder
Does the patient have any other illnesses that may predispose to a bleeding disorder?	e.g. liver disease
Is the patient taking any anticoagulants or bone marrow suppressants?	such agents predispose to bleeding

Fig. 9.4 Questions to ask when considering differential diagnoses of bleeding.

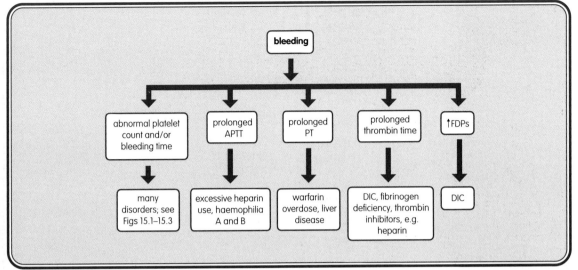

Fig. 9.5 Diagnostic algorithm for bleeding. (APTT, activated partial thromboplastin time; DIC, disseminated intravascular coagulation; FDPs, fibrin degradation products; PT, prothrombin time.)

- What questions would you ask and which investigations would you perform in a patient with anaemia, and why?
- What questions would you ask and which investigations would you perform in a patient presenting with bleeding, and why?

10. Clinical Examination

The clinical examination of a patient may be broken down into four important stages. It is customary, and essential for finals, to approach these in a consistent and systematic order. These stages are:

- *Inspection*—many important signs may be observed simply by looking at the patient carefully.
- *Palpation*—'laying hands on the patient'—this includes feeling for tenderness, masses, enlarged organs, pulses, joint mobility, chest expansion, etc.
- *Percussion*—this involves placing a finger on the patient's skin and tapping it with the index finger of the other hand to illicit a sound that may be resonant or dull, depending on the underlying tissue.
- *Auscultation*—using your stethoscope to listen to the heart, lungs, arteries (for bruits), and abdomen (for bowel sounds).

The signs of immunological and haematological disease manifest themselves in many body systems. It is sensible to examine the different parts of the body in a consistent order: the commonest approach is to start at the hands, working through radial pulses and blood pressure, to the face, and then down the body to the neck, thorax, abdomen, and lower limbs.

It should be noted that this chapter is not designed to be an exhaustive list of physical signs: rather, the more common signs that may be relevant to diseases of the blood and the immune system are highlighted. You should be aware that these signs may have other causes. It is essential, therefore, to interpret all examination findings in the context of a full clinical history.

Important points to note on general inspection	
Sign	**Diagnostic inferences**
thin, wasted appearance (cachexia)	malignancy, especially lymphomas—*but also consider malnutrition or malabsorption*
pallor	anaemia
yellow discoloration (jaundice)	haemolysis—*but also consider liver or biliary-tract abnormalities*
ruddy complexion (plethoric appearance)	polycythaemia
purpura (no blanching on pressure) = petechiae (pinpoint haemorrhages in the skin) and ecchymoses (small bruises)	• with thrombocytopenia—leukaemias (especially acute ones), ITP, DIC, drugs, post transfusion, thrombotic thrombocytopenic purpura, haemolytic–uraemic syndrome • without thrombocytopenia—purpura simplex, senile purpura, hereditary haemorrhagic telangiectasia, Henoch-Schönlein purpura, drugs
extensive bruising	defects of the coagulation cascade
respiratory distress	anaemia—*but also consider respiratory or cardiovascular disease*

Fig. 10.1 Important points to note on general inspection. (ITP, idiopathic thrombocytopenic purpura; DIC, disseminated intravascular coagulation.)

In finals, it is important to be overt when observing the patient—just like looking in the rear-view mirror during a driving test—as quite a few marks can be picked up here.

General inspection

Before you do anything else, introduce yourself to the patient. Always start your examination by standing at the end of the bed and observing the patient. Many aspects of general inspection can be achieved by regarding the patient as you take the clinical history.

Fig. 10.1 outlines the major points to look for on general inspection, and highlights those with relevance to diseases of the blood or immune system.

The hands and arms

After inspecting the patient, it is customary to begin the examination at the hands, where many important signs can be found (Fig. 10.2). Inspect the nails, palms, and muscles of the hands. Are they warm and well-perfused? Make sure you check *both* hands.

Work your way up the arm, checking radial pulse rate, rhythm, and character. Then measure the blood pressure—in finals the examiners may let you skip this, *but it is essential that you state this is what you would have done.* After this, it is a good idea to move to the head and work your way down the body.

The head and neck

Start at the top and work down. Briefly inspect the scalp for anything obvious. Gently pull down the lower eyelid (warn the patient you are about to do this) and inspect the conjunctiva. Inspect the lips and tongue, then palpate for lymph nodes of the head and neck. Check the jugular venous pressure (JVP) and the trachea (for deviation) before continuing on to the thorax.

Fig. 10.3 highlights the important findings of the head and neck that may be relevant to immunological or haematological pathology.

Examination of the limbs		
Examination	**Sign**	**Diagnostic inferences/comment**
inspection of nails	spoon-shaped nails (koilonychia)	iron deficiency—*but also consider syphilis*
	transverse furrows (Beau's lines)	severe illness arrests nail growth
	nail-fold infarcts	vasculitis
	periungual warts (around nail-fold)	common in the immunosuppressed
inspection of nail-beds	nail-bed pallor	anaemia
examination of joints	red, hot, swollen joints; look for signs of joint destruction (subluxation, deviation, etc.) and rheumatoid nodules	rheumatoid arthritis, or other autoimmune disease with joint involvement; haemarthroses in haemophilia; infarcts in heads of long bones associated with sickle cell disease

Fig. 10.2 Examination of the limbs.

The thorax

Inspect the chest for scars, skin lesions, chest wall deformities, and abnormalities of breathing. Examine the heart: palpate the apex beat and check the precordium for heaves and thrills; auscultate the heart. Examine the respiratory system: assess expansion and tactile vocal fremitus (TVF; say '99'); percuss the chest; auscultate for breath sounds.

The abdomen

Inspect the abdomen for skin lesions, scars, obvious masses, and distension. Ask the patient to raise his or her legs off the bed and cough—this may reveal hernias.

Palpate the abdomen lightly in the nine regions for tenderness and obvious masses, keeping your eyes on the patient's face. Then palpate more deeply and investigate any masses you find. Palpate for the liver, spleen, and kidneys.

Percuss out the liver from above and below (you should always percuss from resonance to dullness) and percuss for dullness in the flanks. Auscultate for bowel sounds and bruits of the renal arteries.

Examine the hernial orifices and external genitalia—again, you may not get this far in finals, *but you must say this is what you would do*. Finally, state that you would perform a PR (per rectum) examination and dipstick the patient's urine for protein, blood, and glucose.

Fig. 10.4 highlights the chest and abdominal findings that may be relevant to diseases of the blood or immune system.

The lower limbs

Check peripheral pulses, joint mobility, and neuromuscular function. Examine the foot for signs of peripheral vascular disease.

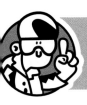

Before you touch the abdomen, ask the patient if it is painful anywhere—if you hurt the patient during finals, you fail!

Examination of the head and neck		
Examination	**Sign**	**Diagnostic inferences**
inspection of skull	bossing of skull	thalassaemia—*but also consider other genetic causes of dysmorphism*
inspection of eyes	pale conjunctiva	anaemia
	reddened conjunctiva	polycythaemia—*but also consider conjunctivitis!*
	yellow conjunctiva (jaundice)	see Fig. 10.1
inspection of mouth	gum hypertrophy	acute myeloblastic leukaemia—*but also consider side effects of drugs, e.g. phenytoin*
	bleeding gums	bleeding disorder, leukaemia—*but also consider gingivitis!*
	white patches	candidiasis in immunocompromised; hairy leukoplakia of HIV disease
palpation for lymphadenopathy	enlarged lymph nodes	discrete, rubbery, non-tender nodes suggest lymphoma; red, tender nodes suggest infection; fixed, hard nodes suggest malignancy

Fig. 10.3 Examination of the head and neck.

Examination of the thorax and abdomen		
Examination	**Sign**	**Diagnostic inferences/comment**
examination of the heart	thrusting apex beat; flow murmur	anaemia—*but also consider valve or myocardial disease*
examination of the lungs	signs of consolidation, e.g. dull to percussion bronchial breathing	atypical pneumonia is common in immunocompromised patients
palpation and percussion for the liver	hepatomegaly	leukaemias, lymphomas, myeloproliferative disorders
palpation and percussion for the spleen	splenomegaly	there are many causes—see p. 143

Fig. 10.4 Examination of the thorax and abdomen.

- What are the four stages of a clinical examination?
- What are the important signs of immunological and haematological disease that may be elicited on clinical examination of the different systems?

11. Further Investigations

HAEMATOLOGICAL INVESTIGATIONS

Common haematological indices are listed in Figs 11.1 and 11.2. The normal ranges represent values for 95% of the population (mean ± 2 SD).

Abnormalities of the peripheral blood film are detailed in Figs 11.3 and 11.4.

Bone marrow examination

Bone marrow can be obtained by two techniques:
- Aspiration.
- Trephine biopsy.

Aspiration of bone marrow involves the insertion of a hollow needle into the sternum or iliac crest. The aspirated marrow is placed on slides, smeared, and stained. Individual cell detail can be assessed well from aspirates.

Trephine biopsy involves insertion of a large-bore needle into the iliac crest. A core of bone and marrow is obtained, which is examined as a histological specimen. These specimens are useful for assessing marrow architecture and cellularity.

The bone marrow findings in some disorders are listed in Fig. 11.5.

Abnormalities of red blood cells		
Parameter	Normal ranges	Diagnostic inferences
red cell count (RCC)	males: $4.4–5.8 \times 10^{12}$/L females: $4.0–5.2 \times 10^{12}$/L	↑—**polycythaemia** (see Chapter 13) ↓—**anaemia** (see Chapter 14)
haemoglobin (Hb)	males: 13–17 g/dL females: 12–15 g/dL	as for RCC
packed cell volume (PCV) or haematocrit = RCC × MCV	males: 0.40–0.51 females: 0.38–0.48	as for RCC
mean cell volume (MCV) = PCV/RCC	80–100 fL (normocytic)	↑ (**macrocytic**)—(A) with megaloblastic erythropoiesis: folate or vitamin B_{12} deficiency; (B) with normoblastic erythropoiesis: physiological (in neonates and in pregnancy), alcoholism, chronic liver disease ↓ (**microcytic**)—(usually also hypochromic), iron deficiency, thalassaemia syndromes, anaemia of chronic disease (can also be normocytic and normochromic)
mean cell haemoglobin (MCH) = Hb/RCC	27–32 pg (normochromic)	↓ (**hypochromia**)—see causes of ↓ MCV
mean cell haemoglobin concentration (MCHC)= Hb/PCV	32–36 g/dL	as for MCH
reticulocyte count	1–2% of circulating red cells $10–100 \times 10^9$/L	↑ (**reticulocytosis**)—haemolytic anaemias; after acute blood loss ↓ (**reticulocytopenia**)—anaemia due to impaired red cell production (see Chapter 14)

Fig. 11.1 Abnormalities of red blood cells.

Coombs' test

Coombs' reagent is a preparation of antibodies, raised in animals, directed against one of the following:
- Human γ-globulin.
- Complement.
- Specific immunoglobulin, e.g. anti-human IgG

The direct Coombs' test

The direct Coombs' test (direct antiglobulin test) is used to detect antibody or complement already bound to the red cells (Fig. 11.6).

A positive direct Coombs' test is found in:
- Autoimmune haemolytic anaemias.
- Alloimmune haemolytic anaemias (haemolytic disease of the newborn and transfusion reactions).
- Drug-induced immune haemolytic anaemias.

The indirect Coombs' test

This is used to detect antibody in the serum (Fig. 11.6). It can be used in the following situations:

- Routine cross-matching of blood prior to transfusion.
- Detection of blood group antibodies in pregnancy.
- Detection of serum antibodies in autoimmune haemolytic anaemias.

In cross-matching of blood, serum from the patient requiring transfusion (patient A) is incubated with the red cells of a potential donor (patient B). Any antibodies in patient A's serum that are specific for patient B's red cell antigens interact with patient B's red cells. Addition of Coombs' reagent then causes agglutination of the red cells as described for the direct Coombs' test

Haemoglobin electrophoresis

This is used in the diagnosis of haemoglobinopathies (Fig. 11.7) and the thalassaemia syndromes.

Abnormalities of white cells and platelets		
Parameter	Normal ranges	Diagnostic inferences
white cell count (WCC)	$4–10 \times 10^9$/L	↑—**leucocytosis**, see Chapter 13 ↓—**leucopenia**, see Chapter 13
neutrophils	$2–7 \times 10^9$/L 40–80% of WCC	↑—**neutrophilia**, see Chapter 13 ↓—**neutropenia**, see Chapter 13
lymphocytes	$1–3 \times 10^9$/L 20–40% of WCC	↑—**lymphocytosis**, see Chapter 13 ↓—**lymphopenia**, see Chapter 13
monocytes	$0.2–1.0 \times 10^9$/L 2–10% of WCC	↑—**monocytosis**, see Chapter 13
eosinophils	$0.002–0.5 \times 10^9$/L 1–6% of WCC	↑—**eosinophilia**, see Chapter 13
basophils	$0.02–0.1 \times 10^9$/L <1–2% of WCC	↑—**basophilia**, see Chapter 13
platelet count	$150–400 \times 10^9$/L	↑—(A) **thrombocytosis** (reactive ↑): haemorrhage, infection, malignancy, chronic inflammation; (B) **thrombocythaemia** (pathological ↑): myeloproliferative disorders, ↓—**thrombocytopenia**, see Chapter 15

Fig. 11.2 Abnormalities of white cells and platelets.

Red cell abnormalities on the peripheral blood film		
Abnormality	**Description**	**Diagnostic inferences**
anisocytosis	increased variation in size (macrocytosis or microcytosis)	see Fig. 11.1 for causes of ↑/↓ MCV
poikilocytosis	increased variation in shape	certain shapes are diagnostic for certain conditions
hypochromia	larger area of central pallor	see Fig. 11.1 for causes of ↓ MCH
spherocytes	small, spherical cells lacking central pallor	hereditary spherocytosis, warm AIHA
sickle cells	crescent-shaped cells	homozygous sickle disease
target cells	cells with central and peripheral dark-staining areas separated by a clear area	thalassaemia syndromes, sickle syndromes, iron deficiency
teardrop cells	teardrop-shaped cells	myelofibrosis and other myeloproliferative disorders
Howell–Jolly bodies	small nuclear inclusions, usually removed by the spleen	postsplenectomy, hyposplenism
Heinz bodies	precipitates of denatured methaemoglobin	glucose-6-phosphate dehydrogenase deficiency
reticulocytosis (polychromasia)	large, bluish cells best seen on supravital staining	see Fig. 11.1 for causes of ↑ reticulocytes
rouleaux	red cells aggregate and stack together	multiple myeloma, Waldenstrom's macroglobulinaemia, cold AIHA

Fig. 11.3 Red cell abnormalities on the peripheral blood film. A normal red cell is described as normocytic and normochromic, and has an area of central pallor.

White cell abnormalities on the peripheral blood film		
Abnormality	**Description**	**Diagnostic inferences**
hypersegmented neutrophils	neutrophil nucleus contains >5 lobes	megaloblastic anaemias
left shift of myeloid cells	immature forms of myeloid cells, e.g. band cells, metamyelocytes	pregnancy, severe infection (leukaemoid reaction), chronic myeloid leukaemia
blast cells	appearance variable—see Fig. 13.6	acute myeloid or lymphocytic leukaemia
Auer rods	rod-like inclusions within cytoplasm of immature neutrophils	acute myeloid leukaemia
smear cells	'smudges' representing disrupted malignant cells	chronic lymphocytic leukaemia
leucoerythroblastic change	nucleated red cells and immature leucocytes	severe haemorrhage/haemolysis, bone marrow infiltration due to myelofibrosis, metastatic cancer, haematological malignancies

Fig. 11.4 White cell abnormalities on the peripheral blood film.

Appearance of the bone marrow in some haematological disorders	
Disorder	**Bone marrow appearance**
iron-deficiency anaemia	absent iron stores from macrophages
megaloblastic anaemias	hypercellular marrow with megaloblasts present; giant metamyelocytes often seen
haemolytic anaemias	hypercellular marrow with erythroid hyperplasia; reduced myeloid/erythroid ratio (usually 2–8)
aplastic anaemia	hypocellular marrow
acute leukaemias	hypercellular marrow infiltrated with blasts
chronic lymphocytic leukaemia	hypercellular marrow with lymphocytic infiltration
chronic myeloid leukaemia	hypercellular marrow with granulocytic and megakaryocytic hyperplasia
multiple myeloma	increased proportion of plasma cells (often abnormal)
polycythaemia rubra vera and essential thrombocythaemia	hypercellular marrow with hyperplasia of all cell lineages
myelofibrosis	early—hypercellularity; late—reactive fibrosis of the bone marrow and reduced haemopoiesis

Fig. 11.5 Appearance of the bone marrow in some haematological disorders.

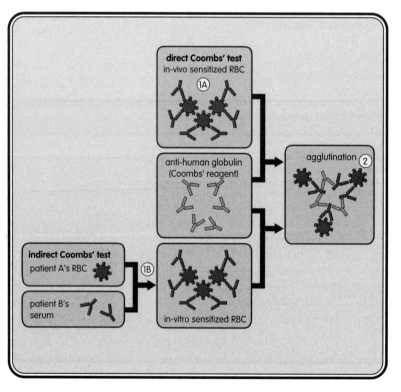

Fig. 11.6 Direct and indirect Coombs' tests. The direct Coombs' test is positive in warm autoimmune haemolytic anaemias where red cells bind to anti-red cell IgG *in vivo* (1A). The red cells do not agglutinate because the IgG antibodies are too small to span the distances between the red cells, but when Coombs' reagent is added, agglutination occurs, indicating a positive result (2). In the cross-matching of blood, patient A's red blood cells are incubated with patient B's serum (1B). Addition of Coombs' reagent causes agglutination of the red cells if there is blood group incompatibility (2).

Cytogenetic analysis

Cytogenetic analysis is the study of structure and function of chromosomes. Certain cytogenetic abnormalities are strongly associated with specific conditions. Important examples in haematology are:

- t (9;22)—this is found in 90% of patients with chronic myeloid leukaemia (the altered chromosome 22 is called the Philadelphia chromosome).
- t (14;18)—this is associated with follicle-centre lymphomas.
- t (8;14)— this is associated with Burkitt's lymphoma.

Lymph node biopsy

Lymph nodes are biopsied for histological examination when malignancy is suspected: for example, demonstration of the Reed–Sternberg cell or its variants against a background of inflammatory cells is required to diagnose Hodgkin's lymphoma.

Other tests are described in the relevant chapters: clotting function in Chapter 6, markers of haemolysis in Chapter 14.

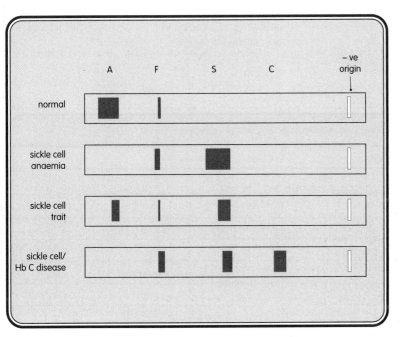

Fig. 11.7 Haemoglobin electrophoresis (normal and in sickle syndromes).

- Summarize the diagnostic inferences that can be drawn from abnormalities of common haematology indices and of the peripheral blood films.
- What is the difference between a direct and an indirect Coombs' test? What do positive results of either test indicate?
- How can haemoglobin electrophoresis be used in the diagnosis of haemolytic anaemias?
- How is bone marrow examined?

INVESTIGATIONS OF IMMUNE FUNCTION

Tests of complement function

The CH$_{50}$ complement screen

This is a haemolytic assay that tests the functional capability of all complement components of the classical pathway.

Decreased complement levels are found in the following:

- Systemic lupus eythematosus (SLE) with glomerulonephritis.
- Myasthenia gravis.
- Hereditary C2 deficiency.
- Severe combined immunodeficiency disease (SCID).
- Acute glomerulonephritis.
- Disseminated intravascular coagulation (DIC).

Increased complement levels are found in the following:

- Physiological overproduction.
- Rheumatoid arthritis.
- Ulcerative colitis.
- Diabetes mellitus.
- Acute rheumatic fever.
- Gout.
- Thyroiditis.

Tests for complement proteins and their inhibitors

Antibodies specific for complement components and their inhibitors are used. Thus, levels can be measured using a variety of methods, including enzyme-linked immunosorbent assay (ELISA). The consequences of deficiency of complement proteins and their inhibitors are outlined in Fig. 11.8.

Clinical manifestations of complement deficiency	
Deficient complement component or inhibitor	**Clinical manifestations**
classical pathway	
C1q, C1r, C1s	SLE, pyogenic infections
C2	SLE, glomerulonephritis, pyogenic infections
alternative pathway	
properdin, factor B, factor D	pyogenic infections, especially *Neisseria* spp.
membrane-attack complex (MAC)	
C5–8	*Neisseria* infections, pyogenic infections
C9	none
both pathways	
↓C3 and ↓C4	SLE, glomerulonephritis, rheumatoid arthritis with vasculitis
↓C3 and normal C4	membranoproliferative glomerulonephritis, paroxysmal nocturnal haemoglobinuria, DIC
regulatory components	
C1 inhibitor	hereditary angioedema, acquired angioedema due to SLE
factor I	pyogenic infections
factor H	haemolytic–uraemic syndrome
DAF, HRF, CD59	paroxysmal nocturnal haemoglobinuria

Fig. 11.8 Clinical manifestations of complement deficiency.

Tests of phagocytic function
These are listed in Fig. 11.9.

Tests of humoral immunity
These are shown in Fig. 11.10

Tests of cell-mediated immunity
These are detailed in Fig. 11.11.

Tests of phagocytic function		
Test	**Description**	**Diagnostic inference**
white cell count and morphology	see Chapter 13	see Chapter 13
nitroblue tetrazolium (NBT) reduction test	NBT is a blue dye that can be reduced by neutrophils subsequent to the metabolic burst—this test assesses the ability of neutrophils to carry out intracellular killing	failure of NBT reduction indicates inability to generate hydrogen peroxide or superoxide: chronic granulomatous disease
tests for degranulation	neutrophils placed in a suspension are unable to ingest fixed γ-globulins and therefore discharge lysosomal enzymes in an attempt at frustrated phagocytosis—the rate of release of lysosomal enzymes is taken as a measure of degranulation	chronic granulomatous disease

Fig. 11.9 Tests of phagocytic function.

Tests of humoral immunity		
Test	**Description**	**Diagnostic inference/comment**
B cell surface markers	monoclonal antibodies detect specific surface markers	e.g. CD19 and CD20 are found on all mature B cells; CD5 is present in some B cell tumours, especially CLL
B cell count	anti-κ and anti-λ antibodies allow measurement of B cell numbers	↑ in bacterial and viral infections
protein electrophoresis/paraprotein measurement	see Chapter 7	see Chapter 7
autoantibody levels	measured using radioimmunoassay and enzyme-linked immunoassay	antinuclear antibody—SLE antimitochondrial antibody—primary biliary cirrhosis and chronic active hepatitis antiparietal cell antibody—pernicious anaemia antithyroglobulin antibody—Hashimoto's thyroiditis anti-AChR antibody—myasthenia gravis
haemagglutination	red blood cells mixed with anti-A and anti-B IgM antibodies—agglutination occurs if A or if B antigens are present; same principle used to determine Rh status	determination of blood groups; gives general indication of IgM production

Fig. 11.10 Tests of humoral immunity.

Tests of cell-mediated immunity		
Test	**Description**	**Diagnostic inference/comment**
skin tests	antigen introduced: • intradermally (Mantoux test) • on a skin patch • via skin-prick	hypersensitivity types I, III, and IV can be assessed
CD4 and CD8 values	direct immunofluorescence performed with fluorochrome-labelled immunoglobulins can be used to estimate T cell subset populations	CD4/CD8 ratio decreased in AIDS (↓ CD4) and other viral infections (↑ CD8); CD8 numbers increase transiently in viral infections
mitogen responses	phytohaemagglutinin (PHA) and concanavalin A (Con A) are T cell mitogens; pokeweed mitogen is a B cell mitogen (T-cell-dependent)	useful in monitoring function in congenital defects or during immunosuppressive therapy

Fig. 11.11 Tests of cell-mediated immunity.

- List the tests of complement function.
- Summarize the tests of phagocytic function.
- List the tests of humoral immunity.
- Summarize the tests of cell-mediated immunity.

IMAGING OF NORMAL AND ABNORMAL BLOOD CELLS

Peripheral blood film

Examination of a peripheral blood film is one of the simplest haematological investigations, yet it provides a significant amount of information, provided the film is properly made and sytematically examined. Films are prepared on glass slides, and it is essential that they are evenly spread. They are then dried and stained, most often with a Romanovsky stain.

Normal blood cells

Normal peripheral blood films are shown in Figs 11.12–11.18.

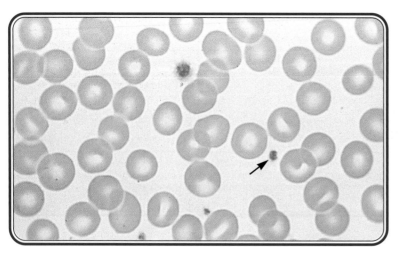

Fig. 11.12 Normal red cells and platelets. Normal mature red blood cells are fairly uniform in size and shape. Most are round, with an average diameter of 7.2 μm, although they can be easily distorted. The cells in this smear show a typical central pallor, indicative of their biconcave morphology. The small, irregular, intensely stained cells are platelets (arrow). (Courtesy of Professor Victor Hoffbrand and Dr John Petit.)

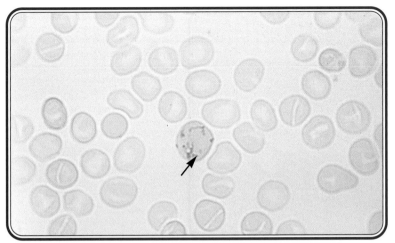

Fig. 11.13 Reticulocytes in normal blood. Supravital staining of a blood film, using new methylene blue, shows precipitated RNA (arrow) in a reticulocyte. Reticulocytes are precursors to mature red blood cells, and account for 1–2% of circulating red cells. A high reticulocyte count is suggestive of haemolytic anaemia or acute haemorrhage. (Courtesy of Professor Victor Hoffbrand and Dr John Petit.)

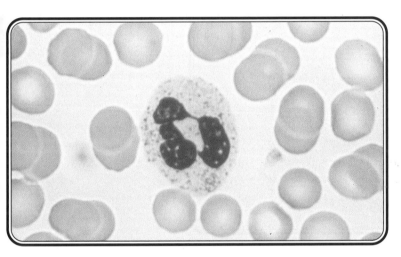

Fig. 11.14 Normal neutrophil. The nucleus is characteristically multilobed, the lobes being connected by strands of chromatin. Most neutrophils have three lobes, as in this case, but up to five may be seen. The cytoplasm contains fine granules. (Courtesy of Professor Victor Hoffbrand and Dr John Petit.)

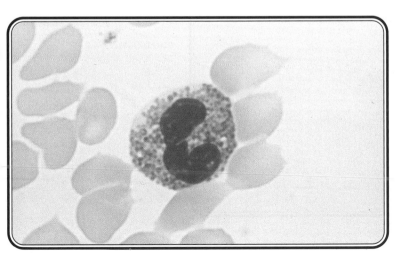

Fig. 11.15 Normal eosinophil. Eosinophils are generally slightly larger than neutrophils. The nucleus is typically bilobed and the cytoplasm contains coarser granules than those seen in the neutrophil in Fig. 11.14. (Courtesy of Professor Victor Hoffbrand and Dr John Petit.)

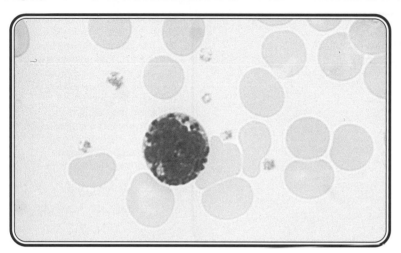

Fig. 11.16 Normal basophil. Basophils are the least common of the circulating white blood cells. In a typical basophil, the nucleus is lobed and the lobes are folded in on one another. Cytoplasmic granules are very coarse and often obscure the nucleus, as in this case. (Courtesy of Professor Victor Hoffbrand and Dr John Petit.)

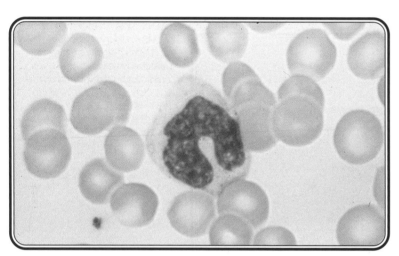

Fig. 11.17 Normal monocyte. Monocytes are the largest of all the circulating white blood cells. In a typical monocyte, the nucleus is folded or convoluted, but not segmented. The cytoplasm contains very fine granules. (Courtesy of Professor Victor Hoffbrand and Dr John Petit.)

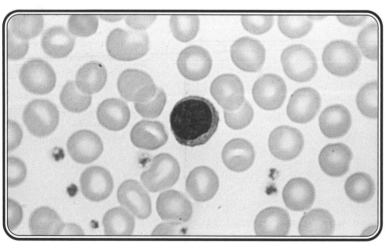

Fig. 11.18 Normal lymphocyte. Lymphocytes are small cells (approximately 9 μm in diameter) with a thin rim of cytoplasm; occasionally, they contain azurophilic granules. (Courtesy of Professor Victor Hoffbrand and Dr John Petit.)

Blood cells in disease

Peripheral blood films can be used in the diagnosis of haematological disease, for example:

- Iron-deficiency anaemia (Fig. 11.19).
- Hereditary spherocytosis (Fig. 11.20).
- Sickle cell anaemia (Fig. 11.21).
- Multiple myeloma (Fig. 11.22).

The concept of right shift is illustrated in Fig. 11.23.

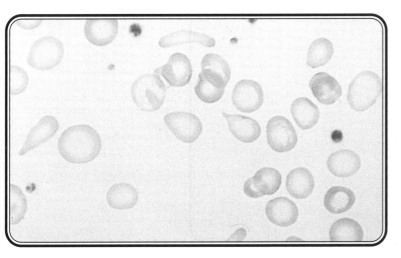

Fig. 11.19 Iron-deficiency anaemia. Red blood cells are typically hypochromic (lightly stained) and microcytic (small cells). (Courtesy of Professor Victor Hoffbrand and Dr John Petit.)

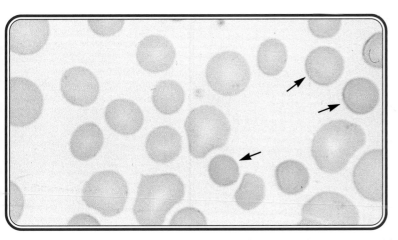

Fig. 11.20 Hereditary spherocytosis. Spherocytes (arrows) are less disc-shaped than normal red blood cells, and are usually smaller and thicker. They are spherical only in extreme instances. In this case, the spherocytosis is due to a genetic defect in a component of the cell cytoskeleton. (Courtesy of Professor Victor Hoffbrand and Dr John Petit.)

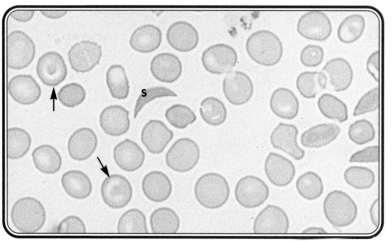

Fig. 11.21 Sickle cell anaemia. Sickled cells vary in shape, from sickles (S), to oat-shaped cells, to elliptical forms. Target cells (arrows) are often seen in blood films of patients with this disorder. (Courtesy of Professor Victor Hoffbrand and Dr John Petit.)

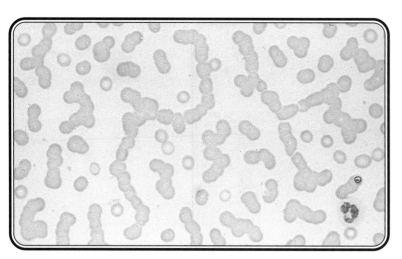

Fig. 11.22 Multiple myeloma. Red cell rouleaux are present. Rouleaux form when there is an increased concentration of high molecular weight proteins, especially immunoglobulins, in plasma. In multiple myeloma, a monoclonal immunoglobulin, a monoclonal light chain (a Bence Jones protein) or both, are secreted by plasma cells and are found in the plasma and urine. (Courtesy of Professor Victor Hoffbrand and Dr John Petit.)

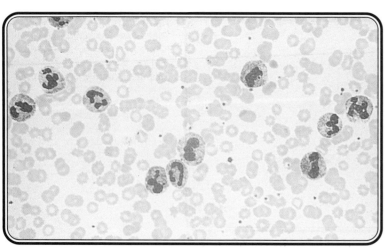

Fig. 11.23 Right shift. Using the neutrophil with its three-lobed nucleus as a marker of normal maturation of granulocytes, a shift to the left or right can be seen. Band forms are evident in this peripheral blood film. The right shift was due to abdominal sepsis. (Courtesy of Professor Victor Hoffbrand and Dr John Petit.)

Bone marrow smear

Bone marrow smears allow examination of the stages of haemopoiesis. Bone marrow aspiration is often the most useful technique diagnostically, but trephine biosy is required when the architecture of the marrow is to be examined. Bone marrow smears are usually stained with Romanovsky dyes, but Perls' Prussian blue may be used to detect iron in macrophages.

Normal bone marrow

Fig. 11.24 shows a normal bone marrow smear.

Lymph node biopsy

A lymph node biopsy from a patient with Hodgkin's lymphoma is shown in Fig. 11.25.

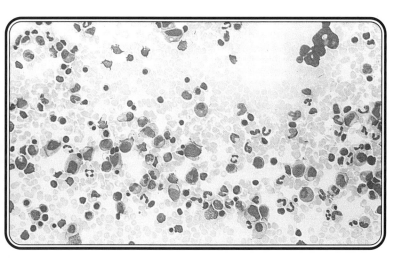

Fig. 11.24 Normal bone marrow smear. Haemopoietic cells and supporting reticuloendothelial cells are visible. (Courtesy of Professor Victor Hoffbrand and Dr John Petit.)

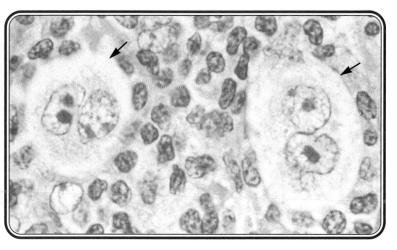

Fig. 11.25 Hodgkin's lymphoma. This lymph node biopsy shows two binucleate Reed–Sternberg cells (arrows). (Courtesy of Professor Victor Hoffbrand and Dr John Petit.)

117

Radiological investigations

Fig. 11.26 shows the radiograph of the skull of a patient with multiple myeloma.

The skull radiograph of a child with thalassaemia major is illustrated in Fig. 11.27.

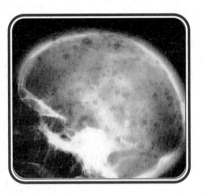

Fig. 11.26 Radiograph of the skull of a man with multiple myeloma. The 'punched-out' lytic lesions are characteristic and are always asymptomatic. (Courtesy of Dr M Makris.)

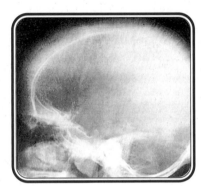

Fig. 11.27 Skull radiograph of a child with thalassaemia major. The 'hair-on-end' appearance is pathogno-monic. It is caused by extramedullary haemopoiesis. (Courtesy of Dr M Makris.)

- Describe the appearances of normal blood cells as seen on a peripheral blood film.
- Give examples of how the peripheral blood film can be used in diagnosis of disease.

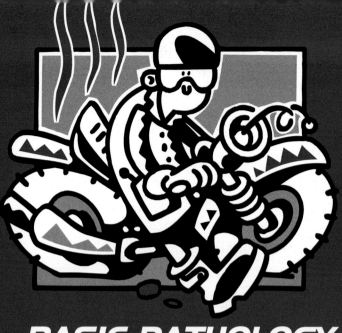

BASIC PATHOLOGY

12. Disorders of Immunity   121

13. Disorders of White Cells, Lymph Nodes, and the Spleen   133

14. Disorders of Red Cells   145

15. Disorders of Haemostasis   155

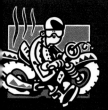

12. Disorders of Immunity

AUTOIMMUNE DISEASE

Autoimmune disease may be organ-specific or systemic.

Systemic diseases

Systemic lupus erythematosus

In systemic lupus erythematosus (SLE), autoantibodies may be directed against DNA, histone proteins, red blood cells, platelets, leucocytes, and clotting factors.

Incidence

The incidence in women aged 20–60 years is 1 in 700. The female:male ratio is 9:1.

Aetiology

The aetiology is unknown, but the vast array of autoantibodies present indicates that SLE is caused by the breakdown of self-tolerance, resulting in profound abnormalities of B and T cells (see Chapter 4).

Genetic factors predispose to the disease. There is an association with HLA-DR2 and HLA-DR3 and the identical twin of a patient with SLE has a 30% chance of developing the disease and first degree relatives have a 5% chance. Deficiencies of complement proteins, especially C2 or C4, are present in 10% of SLE patients but in only 1% of the normal population. Other relevant aetiological factors include drugs such as hydralazine and exposure to ultraviolet light.

Rheumatoid arthritis

Rheumatoid arthritis (RA) is a chronic systemic disease which primarily involves the joints, resulting in inflammation of the synovium and destruction of the articular cartilage (Fig. 12.1). The disease initially affects the small joints of the hands and feet symmetrically, later spreading to the larger joints.

Incidence

RA affects approximately 1–2% of the world's population and is most common betwen the ages of 30 and 55 years. The female:male ratio is 3:1.

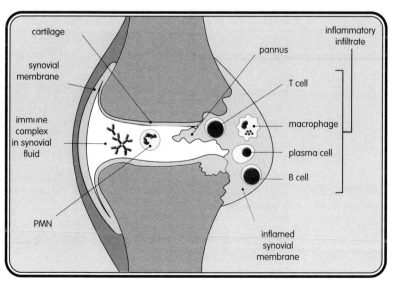

Fig. 12.1 Rheumatoid joint showing pannus formation and cartilage destruction. The synovial membrane is infiltrated by inflammatory cells, and hypertrophies and forms granulation tissue known as 'pannus'. This eventually erodes the articular cartilage and bone. (PMN, polymorphonuclear neutrophil.)

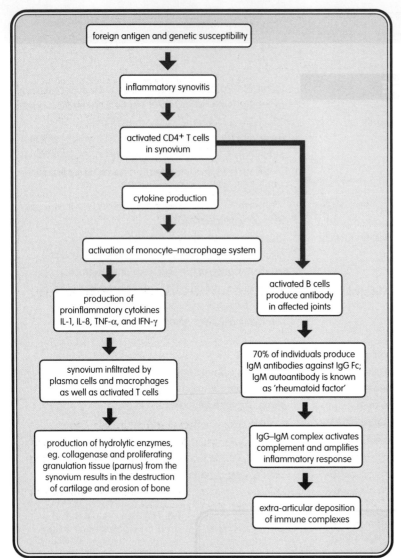

Fig. 12.2 Immunopathogenesis of rheumatoid arthritis (RA). Extra-articular deposition of immune complexes produces some of the systemic manifestations of RA, e.g. vasculitis. Other extra-articular features include rheumatoid nodules, splenomegaly, lymphadenopathy, pericarditis, pulmonary fibrosis and sleritis.

Within the figure:

- foreign antigen and genetic susceptibility
- inflammatory synovitis
- activated CD4⁺ T cells in synovium
- cytokine production
- activation of monocyte–macrophage system
- production of proinflammatory cytokines IL-1, IL-8, TNF-α, and IFN-γ
- synovium infiltrated by plasma cells and macrophages as well as activated T cells
- production of hydrolytic enzymes, eg. collagenase and proliferating granulation tissue (parnus) from the synovium results in the destruction of cartilage and erosion of bone
- activated B cells produce antibody in affected joints
- 70% of individuals produce IgM antibodies against IgG Fc; IgM autoantibody is known as 'rheumatoid factor'
- IgG–IgM complex activates complement and amplifies inflammatory response
- extra-articular deposition of immune complexes

Aetiology

Approximately 70% of RA patients carry either the HLA-DR4 or the HLA-DR1 haplotype or both and there is an increased incidence in those with a family history (5–10%). It has been hypothesized that these and other genetic determinants may render a host susceptible to foreign antigens such as bacteria (e.g. mycobacteria) or viruses (e.g. Epstein–Barr virus), leading to the development of the disease. The immunopathogenesis of RA is outlined in Fig. 12.2. Some other systemic autoimmune diseases are listed in Fig. 12.3.

Organ-specific autoimmune disease
Hashimoto's thyroiditis

Hashimoto's thyroiditis is a disease of unknown aetiology that ultimately results in the destruction of the

Disease	Main characteristics
Sjögren's syndrome	reduced lacrimal and salivary gland secretion, causing dry eyes and mouth
Reiter's syndrome	clinically defined by triad of arthritis, urethritis, and conjunctivitis
systemic sclerosis	increased collagen deposition in skin; usually runs indolent course, but eventual involvement of internal organs occurs in most patients
polyarteritis nodosa (PAN)	usually occurs in middle-aged men (M:F ratio of 3:1); necrotizing vasculitis of small-to-medium-sized arteries (e.g. renal and coronary arteries), often associated with hepatitis B antigen; may be secondary to immune complex deposition
mixed connective tissue disease (MCTD)	features of SLE, RA, scleroderma, and polymyositis; may not be a distinct entity; more prevalent in women than in men

Fig. 12.3 Main characteristics of systemic autoimmune diseases.

thyroid gland. Marked lymphocytic infiltration (mainly B cells and CD4$^+$ T cells) of the thyroid gland is accompanied by migration of large numbers of macrophages and plasma cells, resulting in the formation of lymphoid follicles and germinal centres within the thyroid. Autoantibody production against thyroid antigens such as thyroglobulin and thyroid peroxidase interferes with thyroid hormone production, resulting in hypothyroidism.

Incidence
Middle-aged females are most commonly affected (female:male ratio of 5:1). The disease is associated with HLA-DR5 and HLA-DR3 haplotypes and with other autoimmune diseases such as SLE, Graves' disease, and RA.

Graves' disease
The aetiology of Graves' disease is unknown. The disease is characterized by hyperthyroidism: this is thought to arise as a result of IgG autoantibody production against parts of the thyroid stimulating hormone (TSH) receptor. Clinical features include ophthalmopathy and pretibial dermopathy.

Incidence
Graves' disease affects 1–2% of females. The female:male ratio is 5:1. There is a strong association with HLA-DR3 in Caucasians and with HLA-Bw35 and HLA-Bw46 in Asians. Graves' disease may be associated with other autoimmune disorders such as Hashimoto's thyroiditis and RA.

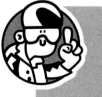

As well as being a systemic autoimmune disorder, rheumatoid arthritis is a very good example of a chronic inflammatory disease, and is therefore twice as likely to come up in exams!

Insulin-dependent diabetes mellitus

This disorder occurs due to destruction of the insulin-producing β cells of the islets of Langerhans of the pancreas.

Incidence

One in 300 people in Europe and the USA are affected. An autoimmune aetiology is suspected. Over 90% of patients with the disease carry either HLA-DR3 or HLA-DR4 or both. Fig. 12.4 outlines the immunopathogenesis.

Some other organ-specific diseases are listed in Fig. 12.5.

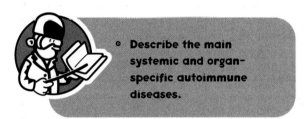

○ **Describe the main systemic and organ-specific autoimmune diseases.**

DISEASES OF IMMUNE DEFICIENCY

Immunodeficiency disorders can be classified as primary or secondary.

Primary immunodeficiencies

These disorders are due to intrinsic defects of the immune system and are often inherited.

Deficiencies of humoral immunity

The disorders caused by deficiencies in humoral immunity are summarized in Fig. 12.6.

Deficiencies of cell-mediated immunity

The causes and features of these disorders are summarized in Fig. 12.7.

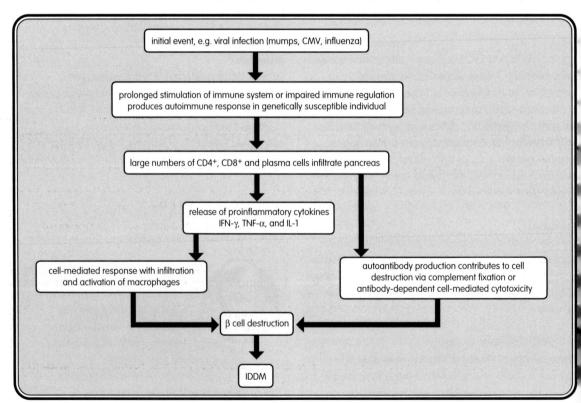

Fig. 12.4 Immunopathogenesis of insulin-dependent diabetes mellitus (IDDM). (CMV, cytomegalovirus.)

Main characteristics of organ-specific autoimmune diseases	
Disease	**Main characteristics**
myasthenia gravis	muscle weakness and fatiguability from impaired neuromuscular transmission; IgG autoantibodies to acetylcholine receptor (AChR) on postsynaptic membrane disrupt transmission by promoting AChR endocytosis and destruction; 70% of patients have thymic hyperplasia, 10% have thymic tumour
Goodpasture's syndrome	clinical features include pulmonary haemorrhage and acute glomerulonephritis; autoantibodies directed against type IV collagen in basement membrane of pulmonary alveoli and glomerular capillaries; peak incidence is in men in their mid-20s
pernicious anaemia	see Chapter 14
AI haemolytic anaemia	see Chapter 14
AI thrombocytopenia	see Chapter 14
AI orchitis	granulomas and immune complexes present within testicular tubules
primary biliary cirrhosis	progressive destruction of intrahepatic bile ducts, eventual cirrhosis and liver failure; antimitochondrial antibodies in 90% of patients; most common in middle-aged women
ulcerative colitis	unknown aetiology; inflammation of colonic mucosa and submucosa

Fig. 12.5 Main characteristics of organ-specific autoimmune (AI) diseases.

Disorders caused by deficiencies in humoral immunity	
Disorder	**Features**
X-linked agammaglobulinaemia of Bruton	X-linked recessive disorder with defect in B cell maturation, resulting in low or undetectable serum immunoglobulin levels present at 6 months with recurrent pyogenic infections; treated with gammaglobulin injections but still sIgA-deficient and therefore prone to respiratory infections
common variable hypogammaglobulinaemia	heterogeneous group of disorders with normal lymphocyte numbers but abnormal B cell function; late onset (15–35 years) presenting with recurrent pyogenic infections and giardiasis
selective IgA deficiency	B cells expressing IgA cannot mature into plasma cells; occurs in 1 in 700 Caucasians but is rare in other ethnic groups; may be asymptomatic or may produce recurrent infections of the respiratory and gastrointestinal tracts

Fig. 12.6 Disorders caused by deficiencies in humoral immunity. Individuals are susceptible to infections with encapsulated organisms such as staphylococci and streptococci, which classically give rise to pyogenic infections.

Disorders caused by deficiencies in cell-mediated immunity	
Disorder	**Features**
DiGeorge syndrome (thymic aplasia)	intrauterine damage to 3rd and 4th pharyngeal pouches results in failure of development of thymus and parathyroid glands; decrease in number and function of T cells; abnormal facies, cardiac defects, hypoparathyroidism, recurrent infections; treated with fetal thymic transplants
severe combined immunodeficiency disease (SCID)	X-linked recessive (>50% of cases) and autosomal recessive forms; 50% of autosomal recessive cases have deficiency of either adenosine deaminase (ADA) or purine nucleoside phosphorylase (PNP), both involved in purine degradation; toxic metabolites accumulate and inhibit DNA synthesis; very low B and T cell levels; children die by age 2 years unless they receive a bone marrow transplant; ADA deficiency has been successfully treated with gene therapy
Wiskott–Aldrich syndrome	X-linked recessive; normal serum IgG levels, low IgM, and high IgA and IgE; defective T cell function, worsening as patient ages; triad of recurrent infections, eczema and thrombocytopenia.
hereditary ataxia telangiectasia	autosomal recessive; chromosomal breaks in TcR and Ig genes; IgA deficiency; ataxia and oculocutaneous telangetesia

Fig. 12.7 Disorders caused by deficiencies in cell-mediated immunity. Individuals are susceptible to opportunistic infections (infections caused by organisms that are not normally pathogenic in healthy individuals) by organisms such as *Pneumocystis carinii*. T cell help is required for the activation of B cells, therefore a T cell deficiency results in reduced humoral immunity.

Deficiencies of phagocytosis
Disorders caused by phagocytic deficiencies are listed in Fig. 12.8.

Complement deficiencies
Disorders caused by complement deficiencies are listed in Fig. 12.9.

Secondary immunodeficiencies
These are far more common than primary immunodeficiencies. They arise as a result of factors such as:
- Malnutrition (an important cause in developing countries).
- Malignancy, e.g. leukaemias, lymphomas, myeloma.
- Drugs, e.g. corticosteroids, cytotoxic drugs.
- Infection, e.g. tuberculosis, HIV.
- Ageing.
- Splenectomy.
- Malabsorption, e.g. due to inflammatory bowel disease.
- Nephrotic syndrome (immunoglobulins lost via kidneys).
- Burns (immunoglobulins lost through skin).

Transient hypogammaglobulinaemia of infancy
This is a secondary immunodeficiency that is universal. IgG is transferred across the placenta from the mother to the fetus principally during the third trimester. After birth, maternal IgG is catabolized by the infant and gradually declines. Production of antibodies by the infant is not sufficient to compensate for this decline, and so, at 3–6 months of age, there is a period of hypogammaglobulinaemia with increased susceptibility to pyogenic infections.

Human immunodeficiency virus (HIV) and acquired immunodeficiency syndrome (AIDS)
The retrovirus HIV is the causative organism of AIDS. It is estimated that 30–40 million people will be infected with HIV by the year 2000, with 1 million dying of AIDS each year. There are two types:
- HIV-1, which has a worldwide distribution.
- HIV-2, which is confined mainly to West Africa.

HIV-1 infection rates are highest in sub-saharan Africa, but are rapidly increasing in south-east Asia and Latin America.

Disorders caused by phagocytic deficiencies	
Disorder	**Features**
neutropenia	see Chapter 13
leucocyte adhesion deficiency	lack of β_2 integrin molecules (due to defective β-chain) results in impaired leucocyte adhesion and extravasation of phagocytes
chronic granulomatous disease	X-linked (most common) and autosomal recessive forms; lack of NADPH oxidase causes failure of production of oxygen intermediates—this impairs killing of ingested pathogens, which can therefore persist, inducing a type IV hypersensitivity response; non-caseating giant-cell granulomas seen on histology; impaired reduction of nitroblue tetrazolium by endotoxin-stimulated neutrophils

Fig. 12.8 Disorders caused by phagocytic deficiencies. Individuals are susceptible to infections with pyogenic bacteria.

Disorders caused by complement deficiencies	
Disorder	**Features**
deficiency of classical pathway components	tendency to develop immune complex disease
C3 deficiency	prone to recurrent pyogenic infections
deficiency of C5, C6, C7, C8, factor D, properdin	increased susceptibility to *Neisseria* infections
C1 inhibitor deficiency	gives rise to hereditary angioedema

Fig. 12.9 Disorders caused by complement deficiencies. Deficiencies of almost all the complement components have been described.

The structure of HIV-1 is illustrated in Fig. 12.10. Transmission of the virus takes place via three routes:

- Sexual contact.
- Exposure to infected blood, e.g. needlestick injuries (risk of transmission following single exposure is 0.3%), blood transfusions.
- From mother to child (transplacentally, during the birth process, and in breast milk).

The primary infection is often asymptomatic, but may be marked by a glandular-fever-like illness in 15% of individuals. This is followed by an asymptomatic period (median 8–10 years) during which individuals may develop persistent generalized lymphadenopathy. The final phase of the disease is AIDS, which is characterized by:

- A low CD4 count (less than 200 cells/μL).
- A number of opportunistic infections such as pneumonia due to *Pneumocystis carinii*, cryptococcosis, and cytomegalovirus infection.
- Cancers, in particular Kaposi's sarcoma and B cell lymphoma.
- Neurological manifestations due both to a direct effect of the virus itself and as a result of opportunistic infections such as toxoplasmosis.

127

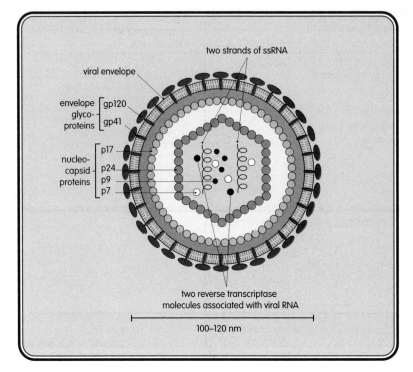

Fig. 12.10 Structure of HIV-1. The envelope glycoproteins gp120 and gp41 are hypervariable. gp120 binds CD4, allowing entry of the virus into the cell. The viral envelope is a lipid bilayer containing both viral glycoprotein antigens and host proteins.

two strands of ssRNA

viral envelope

envelope glyco- proteins [gp120 gp41]

nucleo- capsid proteins [p17 p24 p9 p7]

two reverse transcriptase molecules associated with viral RNA

100–120 nm

The AIDS-related complex (ARC) refers to a collection of symptoms that precede the onset of full-blown AIDS. HIV-2 has lower transmission rates than HIV-1 and runs a more benign clinical course.

Immunology of HIV infection
The gp120 antigen of HIV-1 binds the CD4 molecule on T helper (Th) cells, cells of the monocyte/macrophage lineage, and dendritic cells. Infected monocytes, macrophages, and follicular dendritic cells in lymph nodes are thought to be the major reservoir for HIV. The following changes occur:

- Depletion of $CD4^+$ T cells results in the inversion of the CD4:CD8 ratio (normally 2:1). The CD4 count is a useful prognostic factor (a CD4 count less than 200/μL in an HIV-positive individual is sufficient to diagnose AIDS).

- Defects in T cell function are seen on both in-vivo and in-vitro testing.
- Polyclonal B cell activation occurs, resulting in hypergammaglobulinaemia.
- Neutralizing antibodies directed against the gp120 and gp41 antigens may be generated but are often not protective because of the highly efficient antigenic drift mechanism of HIV.

Laboratory features of HIV infection
These are illustrated in Fig. 12.11.

Screening for HIV infection is performed by using enzyme-linked immunosorbent assays (ELISAs) to detect anti-HIV antibodies. If the ELISA is positive, confirmatory tests must be carried out, e.g. a Western blot, which detects antibodies against HIV proteins. It is important to note that seroconversion may not take

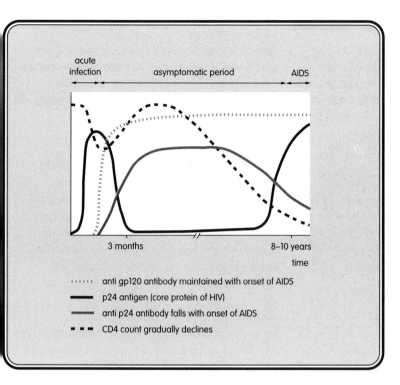

acute
infection | asymptomatic period | AIDS

3 months

8–10 years

time

・・・・・・ anti gp120 antibody maintained with onset of AIDS

━━━ p24 antigen (core protein of HIV)

━━━ anti p24 antibody falls with onset of AIDS

■ ■ ■ CD4 count gradually declines

Fig. 12.11 Changes in antibody and antigen levels during the course of HIV infection.

place until 3 months after infection, hence there is a window period when antibodies will not be detected in the serum. Assays for the p24 antigen or demonstration of the viral genome using the polymerase chain reaction can be used to make a diagnosis in such cases.

In infants, anti-HIV IgG may be maternally derived and can persist for up to 18 months, complicating the picture. Detection of anti-HIV IgA, which does not cross the placenta and is present by 3–6 months of age, or antigen detection may be used to make the diagnosis.

- **Describe the immunological features of the principal primary immunodeficiencies (humoral, cell-mediated, phagocytic, and complement).**
- **What are the causes of secondary immunodeficiency?**
- **Describe the immunology, laboratory features, and diagnosis of HIV infection.**

AMYLOIDOSIS

Amyloidosis represents a number of disorders (Fig. 12.12) that are characterized by the deposition of amyloid, the name given to a heterogeneous group of proteins that share certain physicochemical features. These features include a fibrillar ultrastructure that gives rise to a β-pleated sheet molecular configuration, rendering the proteins resistant to degradation.

Amyloid is deposited extracellularly—often in basement membranes and blood vessel walls—in a wide range of tissues, and has an eosinphilic (pink) appearance in haematoxylin and eosin preparations (H&E). Amyloid can be stained using Congo Red and Sinus Red dye. The former is used as part of a diagnostic test.

Systemic amyloidosis
Primary amyloidosis
Amyloid fibrils known as amyloid light chain (AL) proteins are characteristic. They are derived from immunoglobulin light chains and can be detected in the urine as Bence Jones proteins. Deposition of AL proteins—typically in the heart, kidney, tongue, gastrointestinal tract, and skin—is associated with plasma cell disorders such as multiple myeloma and Waldenstrom's macroglobulinaemia. Primary amyloidosis may also occur as a primary disease, with no apparent lymphoid cell neoplasm.

Reactive systemic (secondary) amyloidosis
This disorder is characterized by deposition of AA-type amyloid protein, which is derived from a precursor known as serum-amyloid-A-associated protein (SAA). Reactive amyloidosis is associated with chronic inflammatory diseases such as RA, bronchiectasis, and osteomyelitis. The kidney, liver, spleen, adrenal gland, and lymph nodes are typically involved.

Dialysis-associated amyloidosis
Up to 70% of patients on long-term haemodialysis are affected. β_2-microglobulin ($A\beta_2M$) is deposited in the joints, synovium, and tendon sheaths, resulting in arthropathy and carpal tunnel syndrome.

Classification of amyloidosis		
	Type of amyloidosis	**Amyloid protein**
systemic amyloidosis	primary	AL (Ig light chain or fragments)
	reactive systemic	AA (serum amyloid A)
	dialysis-associated	$A\beta_2M$
	familial Mediterranean fever	AA
	familial amyloid polyneuropathy	transthyretin
localized amyloidosis	medullary carcinoma of the thyroid	calcitonin-derived
	insulin-resistant diabetes mellitus	amylin
	senile cardiac	transthyretin
	senile cerebral (Alzheimer's)	A4

Fig. 12.12 Classification of amyloidosis.

Hereditary amyloidoses

These disorders are rare and can be divided into further subgroups.

Familial Mediterranean fever

This is inherited as an autosomal recessive disorder and occurs in persons of eastern Mediterranean origin, especially Sephardic Jews and Arabs. Generalized AA-type amyloid is found, especially in blood vessel walls.

Familial amyloid polyneuropathy

This is an autosomal dominant disorder in which a mutant form of transthyretin (a serum protein that transports thyrosine and retinol) is deposited in peripheral and autonomic nerves.

Localized amyloidosis

Amyloid deposition (AL type) is constrained to a single organ or tissue in the absence of precipitating disease. The lungs, larynx, bladder, and skin are most commonly affected.

Amyloid protein deposition may occur in neoplastic or degenerative disorders of endocrine glands (endocrine amyloid). These amyloid proteins are derived from locally synthesized polypeptide hormones or prohormones. For example, a malignant tumour of calcitonin-producing thyroid C cells is known as medullary thyroid carcinoma, and the fibrils deposited are derived from calcitonin. Amyloid deposition may also occur in the islets of Langerhans in association with insulin-resistant diabetes mellitus. The amyloid protein deposited is known as amylin.

Amyloid of ageing

Amyloid deposits may be found in the heart (senile cardiac amyloidosis), where the amyloid protein is derived from transthyretin. Alzheimer's disease is characterized by deposition of an A4 protein (or β-amyloid protein) in cerebral blood vessel walls. The gene encoding this protein has been localized to chromosome 21.

- ○ **Describe the structure of amyloid.**
- ○ **List the various forms of systemic and localized amyloidosis.**

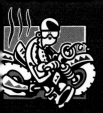

13. Disorders of White Cells, Lymph Nodes, and the Spleen

LEUCOPENIA

Useful definitions

Leucopenia

This is a reduced total white cell count (normal = $4–10 \times 10^9$/L). Leucopenia is usually a consequence of neutropenia (see below).

Neutropenia (granulocytopenia)

This is a reduced total neutrophil count (at age 1 month to 10 years, $<1.5 \times 10^9$/L; at 11–70 years, $<1.8 \times 10^9$/L).

Agranulocytosis

This is a severe reduction in neutrophil count resulting in absence or almost complete absence of neutrophils in the peripheral blood ($<0.5 \times 10^9$/L). It is associated with a substantial risk of infection.

Lymphopenia

This is a reduced total lymphocyte count (normal = $1–3 \times 10^9$/L).

Causes of neutropenia and agranulocytosis

Many different conditions are associated with these disorders.

Inadequate granulopoiesis

This is the reduction or ineffective production of neutrophils in the bone marrow resulting in neutropenia. Causes include:

- Aplastic anaemia—a group of disorders characterized by anaemia, thrombocytopenia, and neutropenia.
- Invasion of the bone marrow by non-marrow elements in leukaemias and lymphomas. Neutropenia is accompanied by anaemia and thrombocytopenia.
- Exposure to certain drugs resulting in haemopoietic stem cell suppression (Fig. 13.1).
- Megaloblastic anaemia due to vitamin B_{12} or folate deficiency—this leads to impaired DNA synthesis, resulting in abnormal granulocyte precursors that are more susceptible to destruction.

Accelerated removal of granulocytes

Causes include:

- Immunologically mediated destruction—this may be idiopathic, secondary to other autoimmune diseases, e.g. Felty's syndrome (rheumatoid arthritis associated with leucopenia and splenomegaly), or due to drug therapy, e.g. chlorpromazine.
- Hypersplenism—this causes splenic sequestration of neutrophils.
- Severe bacterial or fungal infection—this results in increased peripheral utilization.

Drug-induced neutropenia

Drug-induced neutropenia is increasing in frequency. Two mechanisms operate:

- Interference with protein synthesis or cell replication of pluripotent stem cells—this results in generalized bone marrow depression and is a dose-dependent response.

Drugs that may cause neutropenia
analgesic and anti-inflammatory agents
hypnotics and sedatives
antimalarials
diuretics and antihypertensives
anticonvulsants
antithyroid drugs
antibiotics
hypoglycaemic agents

Fig. 13.1 Drugs that may cause neutropenia.

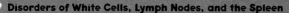

- Immunologically mediated destruction of neutrophils via mechanisms similar to those causing drug-induced haemolytic anaemias—this is not related to drug dose, and neutropenia usually occurs early in the course of the therapy.

Causes of lymphopenia

The causes of lymphopenia are:
- Corticosteroid therapy.
- Trauma or surgery.
- Cushing's syndrome.
- Systemic lupus erythematosus (SLE).
- Hodgkin's lymphoma.
- AIDS.

- Define leucopenia, neutropenia, agranulocytosis, and lymphopenia.
- What are the causes of neutropenia?

REACTIVE PROLIFERATION OF WHITE CELLS

Leucocytosis

Leucocytosis is an increase in the total white cell count ($>11 \times 10^9$/L) and usually consists of raised levels of one leucocyte type with small increases in the other cell lines. An increase in neutrophil levels (neutrophil leucocytosis) is the commonest cause of a leucocytosis. Fig. 13.2 outlines the numerical criteria for raised differential white cell counts.

Causes of reactive white cell proliferation

The diseases associated with the various increases in white cell count are listed in Fig. 13.3.

- What are the causes of leucocytosis, neutrophilia, eosinophilia, basophilia, lymphocytosis, and monocytosis?

NEOPLASTIC PROLIFERATION OF WHITE CELLS

Malignant lymphomas

Lymphomas are malignant neoplasms of monoclonal origin that arise from lymphoid cells. They may originate in the lymph nodes or from extranodal lymphoid tissue, e.g. mucosal associated lymphoid tissue (MALT), spleen.

Malignant lymphomas can be divided into two broad categories:
- Hodgkin's disease (Hodgkin's lymphoma).
- Non-Hodgkin's lymphoma.

A revised European–American classification of lymphoid neoplasms (REAL) has recently been formulated to replace the working formulation and Kiel classification of lymphomas. Tumours are divided into three main categories:
- Hodgkin's disease.
- B cell neoplasms.
- T cell neoplasms.

Hodgkin's disease

Hodgkin's disease (HD) characteristically affects young males in the third and fourth decades of life. Diagnosis requires the presence of the Reed–Sternberg (RS) cell or one of its derivatives in all cases. These pathognomonic cells are typically mixed with a variable inflammatory infiltrate. Disease severity is directly proportional to the number of RS cells found in the lesions and is indirectly linked to the numbers of lymphocytes in the lesions. The RS cell and its variants have been proposed as the malignant

Numerical criteria for raised differential white cell counts	
Cell type	**Levels**
leucocytes	leucocytosis: $>11 \times 10^9$/L
neutrophils	neutrophilia (neutrophil leucocytosis): $>7.5 \times 10^9$/L
eosinophils	eosinophilia: $>0.6 \times 10^9$/L
basophils	basophilia: $>0.05 \times 10^9$/L
lymphocytes	lymphocytosis: $>5 \times 10^9$/L in adults
monocytes	monocytosis: $>1 \times 10^9$/L

Fig. 13.2 Numerical criteria for raised differential white cell counts.

Diseases associated with increases in white cell counts		
Raised cell type	**Associated diseases**	**Examples**
leucocytes	pathological stress, leukaemia	—
neutrophils	bacterial infections	especially pyogenic bacteria
	acute inflammation or tissue necrosis	infarction, surgery, burns, myositis, vasculitis
	neoplasms	carcinoma, lymphoma, melanoma
	myeloproliferative disorders	chronic myeloid leukaemia, myelofibrosis
	metabolic disorders	uraemia, eclampsia, gout, diabetic ketoacidosis
eosinophils	parasitic infestation	malaria, hookworm, filariasis, schistosomiasis
	allergic reaction	asthma, hay fever
	skin disease	pemphigus, eczema, psoriasis, dermatitis herpetiformis
	neoplasms	Hodgkin's disease, metabolic carcinoma, chronic myeloid leukaemia, polyarteritis nodosa (PAN)
	infections	TB, fungal infections
basophils	myeloproliferative disorders	chronic myeloid leukaemia and others
lymphocytes	acute infections	infectious mononucleosis, pertussis, rubella, viral infection
	chronic infections	TB, syphilis
	neoplasms	chronic lymphocytic leukaemia, lymphomas
monocytes	chronic infections and inflammatory diseases	TB, bacterial endocarditis
	neoplasms	lymphomas, myelodysplastic syndromes

Fig. 13.3 Diseases associated with increases in white cell counts.

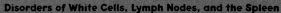

cells of HD. RS cells are binucleated or multinucleated, with prominent eosinophilic nucleoli, giving rise to the so-called owl's-eye appearance.

Classification of Hodgkin's disease

The REAL classification divides HD into five histological subtypes:
- Lymphocyte predominance.
- Mixed cellularity.
- Lymphocyte depletion.
- Nodular sclerosis.
- Lymphocyte-rich classical HD (provisional entity).

Lymphocyte predominance accounts for 10% of cases of HD. The infiltrate consists of large numbers of lymphocytes and histiocytes, interspersed with a few RS cells. This subtype has a good prognosis.

Mixed cellularity accounts for 30% of cases of HD. It is characterized by an infiltrate of histiocytes, plasma cells, and eosinophils. Fewer lymphocytes and more RS cells are present than in the lymphocyte-predominant form of the disease.

Lymphocyte depletion accounts for 10% of cases of HD. RS cells or their variants are present in large numbers in conjunction with relatively few lymphocytes. Lymphocyte depletion has the poorest prognosis of all forms of HD.

Nodular sclerosis accounts for 50% of cases of HD and, unlike other forms of HD, is more common in women. Broad bands of collagen fibres divide the lymph node into nodules containing a mixture of lymphocytes, eosinophils, plasma cells, macrophages, and lacunar cells.

Although histological composition is an important prognostic factor, clinical staging (Ann-Arbor staging) is the most accurate indicator of long-term prognosis in HD.

Ann-Arbor staging is also applied to non-Hodgkin's lymphoma (Fig. 13.4).

All stages are further subdivided depending on the absence (A) or presence (B) of systemic symptoms such as fever, night sweats, and unexplained weight loss.

Non-Hodgkin's lymphomas

Approximately 80% of non-Hodgkin's lymphomas (NHLs) originate from B cells and most of the remainder arise from T cells (Fig. 13.5). The aetiology of NHLs is unknown.

Ann-Arbor staging of Hodgkin's and non-Hodgkin's lymphomas	
Stage	**Sites of involvement**
I	involvement of single lymph node region (I) or involvement of single extranodal site (IE)
II	involvement of two or more lymph node regions on same side of diaphragm (II) or with limited involvement of adjacent extranodal site (IIE)
III	involvement of lymph node regions, including spleen, on both sides of diaphragm (III) and/or limited involvement of adjacent extranodal site (IIIE)
IV	diffuse involvement of one or more extranodal tissues, with or without lymphatic involvement

Fig. 13.4 Ann-Arbor staging of Hodgkin's and non-Hodgkin's lymphomas.

Leukaemias

Leukaemias are neoplastic proliferations of the haemopoietic stem cells within the bone marrow. They are clonal disorders, i.e. they arise from the neoplastic proliferation of a single cell. Leukaemia 'blast' cells replace normal bone marrow and encroach on normal haemopoietic cell development. This leads to:

- Anaemia.
- Neutropenia.
- Thrombocytopenia.

Classification of leukaemia is based on:

- Cell type (lymphoid or myeloid).
- Maturity of leukaemic cells—acute leukaemia involves proliferation of immature cells (blasts) and is rapidly fatal; chronic leukaemia involves more mature cells, and a more prolonged course is characteristic.

Acute leukaemias

Acute leukaemias, characterized by the presence of 'blasts' in the bone marrow and peripheral blood, can be divided into two broad morphological groups:

- Acute myeloblastic leukaemia (AML).
- Acute lymphoblastic leukaemia (ALL).

The French–American–British (FAB) classification further subdivides acute leukaemia into different groups based on their morphology and cytochemistry (Fig. 13.6).

Acute myeloblastic leukaemia

AML increases in incidence with age. It is characterized by the presence of myeloblasts and early promyelocytes, which often contain distinct, rod-like structures in the cytoplasm (Auer rods). Overall long-term survival after treatment is only 30%.

REAL classification of non-Hodgkin's lymphomas
B cell neoplasms
precursor B lymphoblastic leukaemia/lymphoma B cell chronic lymphocytic leukaemia/prolymphocytic leukaemia/small lymphocytic lymphoma lymphoplasmacytoid lymphoma mantle cell lymphoma follicle centre lymphoma—follicular grades I, II, and III extranodal marginal zone B cell lymphoma (low grade B cell lymphoma of MALT type) hairy cell leukaemia plasmacytoma/plasma cell myeloma diffuse large B cell lymphoma primary mediastinal large B cell lymphoma Burkitt's lymphoma
T cell neoplasms
precursor T lymphoblastic lymphoma/leukaemia T cell chronic lymphocytic leukaemia/prolymphocytic leukaemia large granular lymphocytic leukaemia—T and NK cell types mycosis fungoides/Sézary syndrome peripheral T cell lymphomas, unspecified (including provisional subtype—subcutaneous panniculitic T cell lymphoma) hepatosplenic τδ T cell lymphoma (provisional subtype of peripheral T cell lymphoma, unspecified) angioimmunoblastic T cell lymphoma angiocentric lymphoma intestinal T cell lymphoma adult T cell lymphoma/leukaemia anaplastic large cell lymphoma—T and null cell types

Fig. 13.5 REAL classification of non-Hodgkin's lymphomas. (MALT, mucosa associated lymphoid tissue.)

FAB classification of acute leukaemias	
Acute myeloblastic leukaemia	**Acute lymphoblastic leukaemia**
M0—undifferentiated myeloblastic leukaemia	L1—homogeneous population of small lymphoblasts
M1—acute myeloblastic leukaemia without maturation	L2—heterogeneous population of large lymphoblasts with one or more nucleoli
M2—acute myeloblastic leukaemia with maturation	L3—homogeneous population of large lymphoblasts (cells similar to those seen in Burkitt's lymphoma)
M3—acute promyelocytic leukaemia	
M4—acute myelomonocytic leukaemia	
M5—acute monocytic leukaemia	
M6—acute erythroleukaemia	
M7—acute megakaryoblastic leukaemia (rare)	

Fig. 13.6 The French–American–British (FAB) classification of acute leukaemias.

Acute lymphoblastic leukaemia

ALL accounts for 80% of all childhood leukaemias. The peak incidence is at 2–8 years of age. Presentation outside of this range confers a poorer prognosis. In 80% of cases, the blast cells are of B cell origin; in the remainder, they are derived from T cells. ALL is more responsive to therapy than AML, and remission rates of 70% are attained.

Chronic leukaemias

Chronic leukaemias can be divided into:
(i) Chronic myeloid leukaemia (CML)
(ii) Chronic lymphocytic leukaemia (CLL)

Chronic myeloid leukaemia

Chronic myeloid leukaemia (CML), also known as chronic granulocytic leukaemia, accounts for 20% of all leukaemias. The peak incidence is at 20–50 years of age. CML arises from a clonal proliferation of myeloid stem cells. A disease marker, the Philadelphia chromosome, denoting a (9;22) translocation is found in granulocytic, erythrocytic, and megakaryocytic precursor cells in 90% of patients. A hybrid gene, bcr:abl, coding for a protein with the tyrosine kinase activity is formed

and may play a critical role in the development of CML. Median survival is 3–4 years, after which the chronic course of the disease tranforms into an accelerated phase (blast crisis) and rapidly leads to death.

Chronic lymphocytic leukaemia

Chronic lymphocytic leukaemia (CLL) occurs most frequently in people over the age of 60 years and accounts for 2–5% of all leukaemias. CLL arises from a proliferation of neoplastic lymphoid cells (B cells in 95% of cases). On a blood film, leukaemic cells resemble mature lymphocytes, although typical 'smear cells' are also seen. Disease transformation into acute leukaemia does not occur. Median survival is 5–8 years, and treatment is usually aimed at limiting rather than controlling the disease.

Myelodysplastic syndromes

This is a generic term used to describe a group of conditions in which there is ineffective (dysplastic) haemopoiesis in the presence of a normal or hypercellular bone marrow. This results in a trilineage dysplasia:

- Anaemia.
- Neutropenia.
- Thrombocytopenia.

Most patients are elderly males. Approximately 30% of patients progress to AML. Median survival ranges from 1 to 3 years.

FAB classification of myelodysplastic syndromes

Better-prognosis subtypes

These comprise:

- Refractory anaemia—in which the proportion of ring sideroblasts in bone marrow is <15% of total erythroblasts. (Sideroblasts are abnormal erythroblasts containing a perinuclear ring of iron-containing granules.)
- Sideroblastic anaemia—the proportion of ring sideroblasts is >15% of total erythroblasts in bone marrow.

Poor-prognosis subtypes

These comprise:

- Refractory anaemia with excess blasts (RAEB)—5–20% blasts in bone marrow.
- RAEB in transformation—20–30% blasts in bone marrow.
- Chronic myelomonocytic leukaemia (CMML).

Multiple myeloma

Multiple myeloma is a malignant monoclonal proliferation of bone marrow plasma cells at various stages of maturation, probably provoked by excess IL-6 production. Myeloma cells have clonally rearranged immunoglobulin genes and secrete a monoclonal immunoglobulin, a monoclonal light chain (a Bence Jones protein), or both. These monoclonal proteins are known as paraproteins and are found in the serum or urine in 98% of patients. They form a discrete band on the electrophoretic strip (Fig. 13.7).

The incidence of multiple myeloma is 4–6/100 000/year. Most patients are aged 55–65 years, and survival with adequate treatment is 3–5 years. The aetiology is unknown, apart from an inceased incidence related to exposure to ionizing radiation.

Clinical features

Bone destruction is a common feature and is thought to arise as a result of bone resorption induced by the production of osteoclast-activating factor (OAF) by the myeloma cells. Bony abnormalities include diffuse osteoporosis and pathological fractures, especially in the lumbar and thoracic spine and the ribs.

Neurological symptoms usually arise due to the compression of the spinal cord or roots by collapsed vertebrae.

Normochromic normocytic anaemia is present.

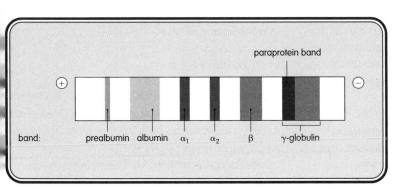

paraprotein band

band: prealbumin albumin α_1 α_2 β γ-globulin

Fig. 13.7 Serum electrophoretic strip of a patient with myeloma. In multiple myeloma, a distinct band in the γ-globulin region is visible. This band is usually made up of IgG, although IgA, Bence Jones protein, IgM, IgD, and IgE may also be found in descending order of frequency.

Repeated infections may occur as a result of suppression of antibody production and a qualitative and quantitative deficiency of neutrophils.

Hypercalcaemia occurs in 10% of cases. This is due to increased reabsorption of bone and is indicative of advanced disease.

Chronic renal failure occurs in 50% of patients. This is caused by:
- Renal tubular obstruction by proteinaceous casts, resulting in atrophy and dilatation of the tubules (myeloma kidney).
- The toxic effect of light chains on proximal renal tubules.
- Light-chain deposition in glomeruli.

Amyloidosis (see Chapter 12) may lead to nephrotic syndrome. An abnormal bleeding tendency occurs owing to the adverse effect of paraprotein on platelets and to coagulation factors.

Solitary myeloma (plasmacytoma)

A plasmacytoma is a solitary tumour found either in the bone or soft tissues, especially the upper respiratory tract. Osseous plasmacytomas usually progress to multiple myeloma. In contrast, with extraosseous plasmacytomas, there is no evidence of dissemination and, after excision and radiotherapy, prognosis is excellent .

Waldenström's macroglobulinaemia

Waldenström's macroglobinaemia is a neoplastic monoclonal proliferation of cells derived from the B cell lineage. As in myeloma, monoclonal immunoglobulin is produced; but unlike myeloma and as in lymphoma, the tumour cells are found in blood, bone marrow, lymph nodes, and spleen. They always secrete an IgM paraprotein (the antibodies are known as macroglobulins owing to their high molecular weight).

The incidence is 3–6/100 000/year and is higher in males than in females. Most patients present between the fifth and seventh decade. Survival averages 2–5 years.

Bone pain and osteolytic lesions are rare, unlike in multiple myeloma. Macroglobulin interference with platelet function and coagulation factors results in a tendency to bleed.

Monoclonal gammopathy of undetermined significance

A paraprotein may be found in 0.1–1.0% of all adults and in 30% of individuals over the age of 70 years without any symptoms or signs of disease. In such circumstances, the term monoclonal gammopathy of undetermined significance (MGUS) is used. MGUS is the most common monoclonal gammopathy. Approximately 20% of patients will progress to one of the conditions described above over a period of 10–15 years.

Langerhans' cell histiocytosis (histiocytosis X)

This is a group of disorders characterized by the proliferation of a specific type of histiocyte (macrophages found in connective tissues) known as the Langerhans' cell, which is usually found in the epidermis. There are three distinct variants:
- Letterer–Siwe disease—this is the most severe form of Langerhans' cell histiocytosis and affects infants and small children under the age of 4 years.
- Hand–Schüller–Christian disease—this is less severe than Letterer–Siwe disease and usually presents before the age of 5 years.
- Eosinophilic granuloma—this has the best prognosis of the three diseases and primarily affects male children and young adults.

Myeloproliferative disorders

These disorders arise as a result of the neoplastic clonal proliferation of multipotent myeloid stem cells, which are capable of following one or more differentiation pathways (Fig. 13.8).

Myeloproliferative disorders encompass:
- Chronic myeloid leukaemia (see p.138).
- Polycythaemia rubra vera.
- Primary thrombocythaemia.
- Myelofibrosis.

Polycythaemia

Polycythaemia is defined as a raised packed cell volume (PCV): in males, to >0.51; in females, to >0.48.

In absolute polycythaemia, the red cell mass is raised. In apparent polycythaemia, the red cell mass is normal, but there is a decrease in plasma volume.

Causes of polycythaemia are listed in Fig. 13.9.

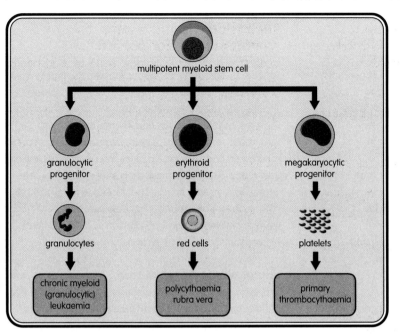

Fig. 13.8 Possible differentiation pathways of multipotent myeloid stem cells and associated myeloproliferative disorders.

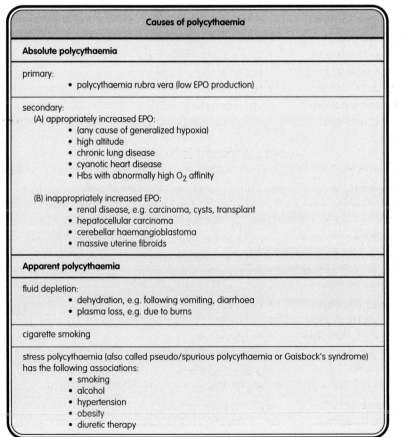

Fig. 13.9 Causes of polycythaemia. (EPO, erythropoietin; see Chapter 5 for its role in regulation of red cell production.)

Causes of polycythaemia
Absolute polycythaemia
primary: • polycythaemia rubra vera (low EPO production)

secondary:
(A) appropriately increased EPO:
    • (any cause of generalized hypoxia)
    • high altitude
    • chronic lung disease
    • cyanotic heart disease
    • Hbs with abnormally high O_2 affinity
 	
(B) inappropriately increased EPO:
    • renal disease, e.g. carcinoma, cysts, transplant
    • hepatocellular carcinoma
    • cerebellar haemangioblastoma
    • massive uterine fibroids

Apparent polycythaemia

fluid depletion:
    • dehydration, e.g. following vomiting, diarrhoea
    • plasma loss, e.g. due to burns

cigarette smoking

stress polycythaemia (also called pseudo/spurious polycythaemia or Gaisbock's syndrome) has the following associations:
    • smoking
    • alcohol
    • hypertension
    • obesity
    • diuretic therapy

Polycythaemia rubra vera

An abnormal clone of stem cells is expanded to give rise to increased numbers of red cells, neutrophils, and platelets. The red cell precursors produced are inappropriately sensitive to erythropoietin (EPO). Haematological findings include:

- Raised PCV and red cell mass (by definition), haemoglobin, and red cell count.
- Raised white cell count (neutrophils and basophils).
- Raised neutrophil alkaline phosphatase.
- Raised platelet count.
- Hyperplasia of erythroid, granulocytic, and megakaryocytic cells in bone marrow.
- Decreased serum EPO.
- Increased plasma urate.
- Increased total blood volume and blood viscosity.

Treatment is by venesection. Other therapies include cytotoxic drugs and irradiation of the bone marrow using ³²P. Some patients develop acute leukaemia or myelofibrosis. The main causes of death are thromboses and acute leukaemia.

Myelofibrosis

The aetiology of myelofibrosis is unknown. It is characterized by the non-clonal (reactive) fibrosis of bone marrow by fibroblasts in conjunction with the proliferation of neoplastic myeloid stem cells, primarily in the spleen. The disease affects individuals from middle-age onwards. Features include anaemia and thrombocytosis (with thrombosis, or bleeding, or both). Massive splenomegaly is common and splenectomy may help. Blood film reveals tear-drop poikilocytosis (tear-drop-shaped erythrocytes). Granulocyte precursor cells and nucleated red blood cell precursors are also found in variable numbers (leucoerythroblastic change). Median survival is 3 years. Approximately 10% of cases transform into AML.

Primary thrombocythaemia

This is a myeloproliferative disorder in which an elevated platelet count is the dominant feature. Platelet counts may be more than 1000×10^9/L (normal = $150–400 \times 10^9$/L). It usually presents after the age of 50 years and is characterized by thrombosis or bleeding (the latter due to abnormal platelet function). There are raised levels of megakaryocytes in the bone marrow. Splenic atrophy occurs in 50% of cases, as a result of microinfarcts.

- What are the differences between non-Hodgkin's lymphomas and Hodgkin's disease?
- List the acute and chronic leukaemias.
- What are myelodysplastic syndromes?
- Briefly describe multiple myeloma.
- What is Waldenström's macroglobulinaemia?
- Briefly describe monoclonal gammopathy of undetermined significance.
- List the myeloproliferative disorders.
- What is the difference between absolute and apparent polycythaemia?
- List the causes of absolute and apparent polycythaemia.
- Summarize the laboratory features of polycythaemia rubra vera and possible modes of therapy.

DISORDERS OF THE SPLEEN

Splenomegaly

Splenomegaly is a frequent clinical finding that may occur in a number of different disorders. The causes of splenomegaly are subject to geographical variation, with the haemolytic disorders predominant in the UK and parasitic causes far more common in tropical countries.

Causes of splenomegaly

Haematological

Haematological causes of splenomegaly include:

- Lymphomas and leukaemias.
- Multiple myeloma.
- Polycythaemia rubra vera.
- Haemolytic anaemias.
- Megaloblastic anaemia.

Infectious

Infectious causes of spenomegaly can be divided into the following:

- Acute—infectious mononucleosis, typhoid fever, toxoplasmosis, bacterial endocarditis.
- Chronic—tuberculosis, brucellosis, syphilis, chronic bacteraemia, histoplasmosis.
- Parasitic—malaria, schistosomiasis, leishmaniasis, echinococcosis.

Portal hypertension

Portal hypertension can give rise to splenomegaly. This can be caused by:

- Liver cirrhosis.
- Cardiac failure (right-sided).
- Hepatic, portal, or splenic vein thrombosis.

Immunological

Immunological causes of splenomegaly include:

- Rheumatoid arthritis.
- Felty's syndrome (hypersplenism in rheumatoid arthritis).
- Systemic lupus erythematosus.

Storage diseases

Storage diseases that result in splenomegaly are:

- Gaucher's disease.
- Niemann–Pick disease.

Hypersplenism

Hypersplenism is characterized by:

- Splenomegaly of any cause.
- Anaemia, leucopenia, and thrombocytopenia, either singly or in any combination.
- Normal cellular or hypercellular bone marrow.
- Correction of the blood cytopenias following splenectomy.

It is thought to be caused by increased sequestration and lysis of blood cells by macrophages in the enlarged spleen.

Congestive splenomegaly

Congestive splenomegaly is caused by persistent venous congestion. Systemic, pre-hepatic, and hepatic causes are the most important ones.

Splenic infarction

Splenic infarction is relatively common and is caused by the occlusion of the splenic artery or its major branches by emboli. It can also be a consequence of local thrombosis caused by sickle cell disease and myeloproliferative disorders. Infarcts may be single or multiple.

Congenital abnormalities

Approximately 10% of the population have accessory spleens. Congenital asplenia (absence of the spleen) is relatively rare and usually occurs in conjunction with other congenital abnormalities.

Rupture of the spleen

Causes include:

- Infections, e.g. infectious mononucleosis.
- Haemopoietic disorders, e.g. myelofibrosis.
- Abdominal trauma, e.g. road-traffic accidents.

There is a lot of detail in this chapter. For an exam, the most important topics are Hodgkin's lymphoma, the leukaemias, polycythaemia rubra vera, and multiple myeloma.

- List the causes of splenomegaly.
- Discuss hypersplenism and its consequences.
- What are the causes of congestive splenomegaly?
- What are the causes of splenic infarction?
- What are the causes of splenic rupture?

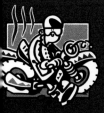

14. Disorders of Red Cells

Anaemia can be defined as a decrease in the total red cell mass, resulting in an inability to maintain tissue oxygenation. This is usually defined by a low blood haemoglobin (Hb) concentration adjusted for age and sex. Changes in plasma volume can also alter the Hb concentration. Anaemias have a variety of causes (Fig. 14.1).

ANAEMIA DUE TO BLOOD LOSS

Acute blood loss
Causes of acute blood loss include trauma, surgery, peripartum haemorrhage, haematemesis, and haemoptysis. Plasma volume is replaced within 1 to 3 days after acute blood loss, but it can take several weeks for the red cell mass to be replenished, during which time the individual is anaemic. Haematological findings include:

- A normocytic, normochromic anaemia.
- A reticulocytosis that peaks 1–2 weeks after the haemorrhage.
- An increase in the number of platelets and neutrophils.
- Neutrophil precursors in the peripheral blood.

Before compensation for the loss of intravascular volume, red cell parameters may be normal, as both plasma and red cells have been lost in their normal proportions.

Chronic blood loss
The most common causes of chronic blood loss are gastrointestinal lesions and menorrhagia. The consequences are those of iron-deficiency anaemia.

Fig. 14.1 Causes of anaemia.

Causes of anaemia	
blood loss	acute blood loss chronic blood loss
increased destruction of red cells (haemolytic anaemias)	(A) hereditary: • membrane defect, e.g. hereditary spherocytosis • metabolic defect, e.g. glucose-6-phosphate dehydrogenase deficiency • haemoglobin defect, e.g. sickle cell anaemia, thalassaemia
	(B) acquired: • membrane defect (paroxysmal nocturnal haemoglobinuria) • immune-mediated, e.g. autoimmune and alloimmune haemolytic anaemias • mechanical trauma • chemicals and toxins • infection • hypersplenism
impaired red cell production	iron-deficiency anaemia megaloblastic anaemias anaemia of chronic disease aplastic anaemia pure red-cell aplasia myelophthisic anaemia chronic renal failure

- **Classify the different types of anaemia by cause.**
- **What are the features of acute blood loss?**

ANAEMIA DUE TO RED CELL DESTRUCTION (HAEMOLYTIC ANAEMIAS)

Haemolytic anaemias are characterized by an increased rate of red cell destruction. The normal marrow can increase erythropoiesis by a factor of six to eight, hence, initially, patients may be in a compensated haemolytic state with no anaemia.

Haemolysis may be intravascular or extravascular.

Extravascular haemolysis is the route by which red cells are normally broken down and occurs in the macrophages of the spleen, bone marrow, and liver (see Fig. 5.6).

Intravascular haemolysis is the destruction of red cells within the circulation. It is characterized by all of the features of extravascular haemolysis (Fig. 5.7), as well as by the following:

- Haemoglobinaemia—Hb is released into the bloodstream.
- Absence of plasma haptoglobulin—Hb binds haptoglobulin to form a complex that is removed by macrophages in the spleen.
- Haemoglobinuria—the Hb concentration exceeds the tubular reabsorptive capacity and Hb is therefore excreted in the urine.
- Haemosiderinuria—proximal tubule cells containing intracellular deposits of haemosiderin derived from the Hb reabsorbed in the kidneys are shed in the urine.
- Methaemalbuminaemia—some of the Hb is oxidized and binds albumin.

Hereditary disorders

The defect is usually intrinsic to the red cell, and morphological abnormalities can often be detected on inspection of a peripheral blood smear.

Membrane defects

Hereditary spherocytosis

Hereditary spherocytosis (see p. 73) is a common autosomal dominant disorder (prevalence of 1 in 5000 in northern Europe). There is an abnormality of one of the cytoskeletal proteins, most commonly spectrin, which results in progressive spherocytosis and reduced deformability of red cells, leading to *extravascular* haemolysis (see Fig. 5.13). Haematological findings include:

- Reticulocytosis.
- Spherocytes on the peripheral blood smear.
- Increased osmotic fragility—when suspended in saline solutions of varying concentrations, spherocytes lyse in less hypotonic solutions than do normal red cells.
- Increased autohaemolysis—when spherocytes are incubated in isotonic sodium chloride, they lyse more readily than normal cells.

Splenectomy will result in a rise in the Hb level. Pneumococcal vaccine must be administered before the operation and prophylactic penicillin is recommended for postoperatively.

Hereditary elliptocytosis

This autosomal dominant disorder is also due to abnormalities of the cytoskeletal proteins and is most commonly caused by failure of the spectrin dimers to form tetramers. It is clinically similar to, but much milder than, hereditary spherocytosis. A high proportion of elliptical red cells are seen on the peripheral blood film.

Metabolic defects

Glucose-6-phosphate dehydrogenase deficiency

Glucose-6-phosphate dehydrogenase (G6PD) deficiency is an X-linked disorder characterized by the lack of the enzyme or by a dysfunctional enzyme (see p.

74). There are over 400 variants of G6PD, two of which account for the vast majority of cases: the African (A) and Mediterranean types. Of these two, the Mediterranean type is clinically more severe, as there is a much greater reduction in enzyme function. Patients are generally asymptomatic and haemolysis is precipitated by factors such as:

- Infection.
- Acidosis.
- Drugs, e.g. primaquine, sulphonamides.
- Fava beans ('favism'—only in the Mediterranean type).

Haemolysis is primarily *intravascular*. During a haemolytic crisis, haematological findings include:

- Reticulocytosis.
- Heinz bodies (precipitates of denatured methaemoglobin) and 'bite' or 'blister' cells (cells that have had Heinz bodies removed upon passing through the spleen) on the peripheral blood film.

In an asymptomatic patient, the peripheral blood film may be normal. G6PD levels are decreased in affected males and carrier females; however, the assay may be unreliable during or immediately after a haemolytic crisis as reticulocytes, which are increased in number during a crisis, have higher enzyme levels than mature red cells. In an acute haemolytic episode, the precipitating factor should be eliminated and circulatory support maintained. There is no specific treatment and patients should avoid precipitating factors.

Haemoglobin defects

Thalassaemias

In thalassaemias, there is a defect in the production of the α or β globin chains. The amino acid sequence of the chains is usually normal, but the rate of synthesis is reduced.

β-Thalassaemia occurs most commonly in Mediterranean countries, South-East Asia, and Africa. There is a partial or complete failure of β globin chain production. The abnormal β-chain genes are denoted β^+ and β^0, respectively.

α-Thalassaemia is most common in South-East Asia and West Africa. There is a deletion of one, two, three, or all four α-globin chain genes.

An imbalance in globin chain production arises, resulting in an excess of α-chains (in β-thalassaemia) or β-chains (in α-thalassaemia), which aggregate within the red-cell precursors, predisposing them to phagocytosis by bone marrow macrophages. Any abnormal red cells that do reach the circulation have a shortened lifespan. The anaemia that results is therefore due to a combination of ineffective erythropoiesis and peripheral red cell destruction, particularly in the spleen.

A number of clinical syndromes are recognized, based on the severity of the anaemia (Figs 14.2 and 14.3). In the β-thalassaemia syndromes, this is determined by whether β^+ or β^0 has been inherited and whether the individual is heterozygous or homozygous. In the α-thalassaemia syndromes, the number of α genes deleted is important.

The β-thalassaemia syndromes		
Clinical syndrome	**Genotype**	**Presentation**
β-thalassaemia major (Mediterranean or Cooley's anaemia)	homozygous ($\beta^0\beta^0$, $\beta^+\beta^+$, or $\beta^+\beta^0$)	onset at 6–9 months, when HbA should have replaced HbF; severe anaemia, jaundice, failure to thrive, hepatosplenomegaly, bony abnormalities, gall stones, leg ulcers, and intercurrent infection
β-thalassaemia intermedia	a variety of genotypes	presents at 1–2 years of age; moderate anaemia, clinically less severe than β-thalassaemia major
β-thalassaemia minor	heterozygous ($\beta^0\beta$ or $\beta^+\beta$)	usually asymptomatic

Fig. 14.2 The β-thalassaemia syndromes.

Investigations and treatment of β-thalassaemia

In *β-thalassaemia major*, β-chain production is severely reduced. Laboratory investigation reveals:

- Microcytic hypochromic anaemia (Hb 2–3 g/dL) and reticulocytosis.
- Basophilic stippling and target cells on peripheral blood film.
- Absence of HbA on Hb electrophoresis.
- High serum iron due to: (i) increased absorption from the gut; (ii) regular blood transfusions.

A 'hair-on-end' appearance is characteristic of the skull X-ray (see Fig 11.27).

Treatment of β-thalassaemia major is by regular blood transfusions (resulting in a problem with iron overload), splenectomy, and/or bone marrow transplantation.

Laboratory investigation of patients with *β-thalassaemia minor* reveals:

- Slightly reduced Hb concentration.
- Microcytic, hypochromic red cells.
- Raised HbA_2 (4–8% of total Hb) on electrophoresis.

Recognition of this syndrome is important as it has implications for genetic counselling (1 in 10 people are affected in Greece and Cyprus). It can also mimic iron-deficiency anaemia, although serum iron, ferritin, and total iron-binding capacity (TIBC) are normal.

Sickle cell syndromes

The sickle Hb (HbS) gene is prevalent in tropical Africa and parts of the Mediterranean, Middle East, and India. Up to 40% of the population may be affected in some areas. It is found in 10% of African Americans.

In HbS, glutamic acid is replaced by valine at position 6 of the β-chain. Deoxygenated HbS is 50 times less soluble than deoxygenated HbA and it aggregates and polymerizes to form long intracellular fibres called tactoids. This is accompanied by elongation of the red cell into the classic sickle shape. Reoxygenation can initially reverse the sickling process, but after repeated episodes of sickling, the red cells eventually become irreversibly sickled.

HbS interacts most effectively with other HbS molecules. The presence of other types of Hb such as HbF and HbA can decrease sickling of the cells because HbS interacts weakly with these types and so fewer polymers are formed. This is why sickle cell anaemia is not manifest until approximately 6 months of age, when HbF levels have fallen, and why individuals with sickle cell trait and sickle cell haemoglobin C disease are asymptomatic or have clinically milder forms of the disease.

There are four important syndromes associated with HbS:

The α-thalassaemia syndromes		
Clinical syndrome	**No. of α genes lost**	**Clinical features**
silent carrier	1	asymptomatic; normal haematological indices
α-thalassaemia trait	2	asymptomatic; mild, microcytic, hypochromic anaemia
HbH disease	3	HbH is composed of β-chain tetramers which are unstable and precipitate, leading to a reduced red cell lifespan; moderate, microcytic, hypochromic anaemia, clinically similar to β-thalassaemia intermedia
hydrops fetalis	all 4	incompatible with life, as functional HbF cannot be produced (death *in utero*); high proportion of Hb Barts* is present in the cord blood

Fig. 14.3 The α-thalassaemia syndromes. *Hb Barts is composed of γ-chain tetramers and may be found in fetuses with any α-thalassaemia syndrome, but its proportion directly correlates with the number of gene deletions.

- Sickle cell anaemia.
- Sickle cell trait
- Sickle cell haemoglobin C disease.
- Sickle cell β-thalassaemia.

Sickle cell anaemia (homozygous for HbS, denoted $\beta^s\beta^s$) is the most serious of these. Clinical features of sickle cell anaemia are listed in Fig. 14.4.

Laboratory findings are as follows:
- Hb 6–9 g/dL.
- Reticulocytosis.
- Sickle cells seen on blood film.
- HbS detected on Hb electrophoresis; no HbA.
- Red cells sickle upon mixing with sodium metabisulphite (sickling test).

- Red cells do not lyse in saponin, unlike normal red cells (solubility test).

Management strategies include:
- Pneumococcal vaccine and penicillin prophylaxis.
- Folic acid supplements.
- Avoidance of factors precipitating infarctive crises.
- Prompt treatment of infection.
- Management of infarctive crises with fluids, analgesia (including opiates), warmth, and antibiotics if necessary.
- Blood transfusions and exchange transfusions when necessary.
- Prevention of iron overload.

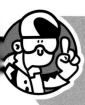

Sickle cell anaemia is a commonly examined topic. Make sure you understand the genetic basis and pathophysiology of the disease, as well as the clinical features and laboratory findings.

Features of sickle cell anaemia	
Feature	**Notes**
chronic haemolytic anaemia	non-deformable sickled cells impact in the microcirculation of the spleen, leading to premature cell death; pigment gallstones are common (see Fig. 5.7)
infarctive or painful crises	sickled cells lodge in small and medium-sized blood vessels; precipitated by hypoxia, infection, acidosis, dehydration, and cold; infarcted metacarpals and metatarsals cause dactylitis (hand–foot syndrome) in children; chronic tissue and organ damage ensues, especially of the bones, lungs, kidneys, liver, and brain
haemolytic crises	usually accompany infarctive crises; ↓ Hb and ↑ reticulocytes
aplastic crises	due to parvovirus infection and to folate deficiency; ↓ Hb and ↓ reticulocytes
spleen	spleen enlarged in young children due to trapped red cells, but shrinks in size and atrophies (autosplenectomy) by ~6 years after repeated vasoocclusive episodes; pre-autosplenectomy patients susceptible to potentially fatal splenic sequestration crises (large volume of blood rapidly trapped in spleen, causing sudden splenomegaly, severe anaemia, and hypovolaemic shock)
infections	risk of overwhelming sepsis in early childhood; in asplenic state, more susceptible to infection with encapsulated organisms, e.g. *Streptococcus pneumoniae*; prone to *Salmonella* osteomyelitis
other complications	priapism, chronic leg ulcers, proliferative retinopathy

Fig. 14.4 Clinical features of sickle cell anaemia.

Sickle cell trait (heterozygous, HbSA, $\beta^s\beta$) individuals are generally asymptomatic. Sickling occurs at very low partial pressures of oxygen that are rarely reached *in vivo*. Both HbA and HbS bands are detectable on electrophoresis and sickled cells are not usually seen on the peripheral blood film. Sickling and solubility tests are positive.

Sickle cell haemoglobin C disease (HbS/HbC, $\beta^s\beta^c$) arises from carriage of two abnormal β genes. It is clinically similar to, but less severe than, sickle cell anaemia. Patients are more susceptible to thrombosis and pulmonary embolism and are more likely to develop proliferative retinopathy.

Sickle cell β-thalassaemia ($\beta^s\beta^0$ or $\beta^s\beta^+$) shares its clinical features with sickle cell anaemia, but its severity is variable and depends on the amount of normal β-chain synthesis.

Both the sickle cell and thalassaemia traits afford some protection against malaria due to *Plasmodium falciparum* and it is thought that the relevant genes are positively selected in areas where malaria is endemic.

Acquired disorders

In acquired disorders, the red cells are usually normal and disease occurs due to factors extrinsic to the cell. An exception to this is **paroxysmal nocturnal haemoglobinuria**, where a red-cell membrane defect is acquired. In this disorder, red cells, white cells, and platelets are deficient in the molecule glycosyl-phosphatidylinositol (GPI). GPI anchors certain proteins to the red-cell membrane, including homologous restriction factor and decay-accelerating factor, two inhibitors of complement (see Fig. 3.31). Lack of these GPI-linked proteins renders red cells more susceptible to complement-mediated lysis, resulting in intravascular haemolysis.

Immune disorders
Autoimmune haemolytic anaemias

In the autoimmune haemolytic anaemias (AIHAs), haemolysis is due to autoantibodies directed against red cells. A positive direct Coombs' test can be demonstrated. There are three types of AIHA:
- Warm AIHA.
- Cold AIHA.
- Paroxysmal cold haemoglobinuria.

Warm AIHA may be idiopathic or secondary to autoimmune disease (especially SLE), leukaemias (especially chronic lymphocytic leukaemia), lymphomas, and drugs (e.g. methyldopa).
  The clinical features are as follows:
- Highly variable symptoms that are unrelated to temperature.
- Splenomegaly almost always present.
- Evans' syndrome is the combination of warm AIHA and idiopathic thrombocytopenic purpura (ITP).

If the disease is secondary, the cause should be eliminated. Patients generally respond well to steroids, but splenectomy is required if they do not. Immunosuppressive therapy may be successful.

Cold AIHA may be idiopathic or secondary to lymphoma or infection (e.g. *Mycoplasma* pneumonia, infectious mononucleosis).
  The clinical features are as follows:
- Symptoms worse in cold weather.
- Acrocyanosis (purplish discoloration of the skin) due to vascular sludging arising from red cell agglutination.
- Raynaud's phenomenon.

Treatment involves elimination of the cause if the disease is secondary. Otherwise, the patient should be kept warm and immunosuppressive therapy considered.
  The laboratory features of warm and cold AIHAs are compared in Fig. 14.5.

Paroxysmal cold haemoglobinuria is characterized by IgG autoantibodies that are specific for the red cell P antigen. These are called Donath–Landsteiner antibodies and are capable of fixing complement, unlike the IgG antibodies of warm AIHA. At low temperatures, antibody and complement bind to the red cells; at higher temperatures, haemolysis occurs.

Features of warm and cold AIHAs		
Feature	**Warm AIHA**	**Cold AIHA**
antibody class	IgG	IgM
antibody specificity	may be specific for Rhesus antigens	may be specific for I or i antigens
optimal temperature for binding to red cell	37°C	< 32°C
red cell agglutination	✗	✓
complement fixation	✗	✓
mechanism of cell destruction	predominantly extravascular	predominantly intravascular
haematological findings	typical of extravascular haemolysis; positive direct Coombs' test for IgG and complement; spherocytes—due to partial phagocytosis of red cells—may be seen on peripheral blood smear (distinguished from hereditary spherocytosis by positive direct Coombs' test)	typical of intravascular haemolysis; positive direct Coombs' test for complement (may be negative for antibody, as antibody detaches from red cells upon passing to warmer central circulation); red cell agglutinates seen on peripheral blood smear, which disperse upon warming slide

Fig. 14.5 Comparison of laboratory features of warm and cold autoimmune haemolytic anaemias (AIHAs).

Alloimmune haemolytic anaemias
These include haemolytic transfusion reactions and haemolytic disease of the newborn (see Chapter 8).

Drug-induced immune haemolytic anaemias
Certain drugs can precipitate haemolysis via immune mechanisms. Examples of such drugs are penicillin and quinine.

Non-immune haemolytic anaemias
These may be secondary to:
- Mechanical trauma; for example, in microangiopathic haemolytic anaemias, the red cells are fragmented due to abnormalities of the microcirculation as in disseminated intravascular coagulation and malignant hypertension.
- Chemicals and toxins, e.g. lead poisoning, some snake venoms.
- Infection, e.g. malaria.
- Hypersplenism.

- **What are the differences between intravascular and extravascular haemolysis?**
- **Summarize the pathophysiology, clinical, and laboratory features of the different types of haemolytic anaemia.**

151

ANAEMIA DUE TO IMPAIRED RED CELL PRODUCTION

Iron-deficiency anaemia

Iron deficiency is the commonest cause of anaemia worldwide. It occurs most frequently in women of reproductive age. Anaemia occurs after iron stores have been depleted.

Causes of iron-deficiency anaemia include:
- Decreased iron intake, e.g. due to poor diet.
- Increased iron requirement, e.g. during pregnancy and lactation.
- Chronic blood loss, e.g. due to peptic ulcer.
- Decreased iron absorption, e.g. after gastrectomy.

The signs and symptoms of iron-deficiency anaemia (Fig. 14.6) are often only apparent when the haemoglobin level drops below 8 g/dL.

The haematological findings are:
- A microcytic, hypochromic anaemia (also seen in the thalassaemia syndromes and chronic disease, but iron deficiency is the commonest cause).
- Reduced serum iron and ferritin.
- Increased serum transferrin and total iron-binding capacity (TIBC).
- Reduced plasma transferrin saturation
- Absence of iron stores demonstrated on bone marrow smear.

Treatment is by correction of the underlying cause, if possible, and oral administration of iron in the form of ferrous sulphate tablets. This must be continued for 4–6 months in order to replenish iron stores. Parenteral iron is used if the patient has malabsorption or cannot tolerate oral preparations.

Megaloblastic anaemias

In megaloblastic anaemias, impaired DNA synthesis results in the appearance of abnormal red cell precursors in the marrow—megaloblasts. These are larger than their normal counterparts and contain relatively large nuclei with more finely dispersed chromatin. Anaemia occurs principally because the megaloblasts are removed by the bone marrow phagocytes (ineffective erythropoiesis).

The most important cause of megaloblastic anaemia is deficiency of vitamin B_{12}, or of folate, or of both. These act as coenzymes in the pathway of DNA synthesis.

Haematological findings include:
- Macrocytic anaemia (macrocytes in peripheral blood owing to megaloblastic erythropoiesis).
- Hypersegmentation of neutrophil nuclei.
- Megaloblasts seen on bone marrow smear.
- Low serum B_{12} levels or reduced red cell folate content (depending on the cause of the anaemia).

Vitamin B_{12} deficiency

Vitamin B_{12} consists of cobalamin bound to a methyl or adenosyl group. It is found only in foods of animal origin and is not affected by cooking. Its absorption in the gut is dependent on intrinsic factor (IF), which is produced by the gastric parietal cells. IF binds vitamin B_{12} in the jejunum, and absorption of the B_{12}–IF complex occurs exclusively in the terminal ileum.

Signs and symptoms of iron-deficiency anaemia	
Signs and symptoms common to other anaemias	**Signs and symptoms specific to iron deficiency**
fatigue	glossitis (smooth, sore, red tongue)
dizziness	
headache	koilonychia (spoon-shaped nails)
shortness of breath	angular stomatitis (cracking at the corners of the mouth)
palpitations	
angina	alopecia
intermittent claudication	pica (unusual dietary cravings for substances such as clay and ice)
pallor	
tachycardia	
flow murmur	
congestive cardiac failure	

Fig. 14.6 Signs and symptoms of iron-deficiency anaemia. The Plummer–Vinson or Paterson–Kelly syndrome is the combination of iron-deficiency anaemia, dysphagia, and a pharyngeal web.

Vitamin B_{12} is stored in the liver. Body stores are large, and the daily rate of loss in urine and faeces is small relative to daily requirements; therefore it takes more than 2 years after the onset of the cause of vitamin B_{12} deficiency before anaemia develops.

Causes of vitamin B_{12} deficiency include:
- Decreased B_{12} intake, e.g. due to a vegan diet.
- Decreased IF secretion, e.g. due to pernicious anaemia.
- Decreased absorption of the B_{12}–IF complex, e.g. terminal ileum disease, as in Crohn's disease.
- Diversion of B_{12}, e.g. due to a blind loop.

Pernicious anaemia

Pernicious anaemia is a chronic atrophic gastritis with a probable autoimmune aetiology and is the commonest cause of vitamin B_{12} deficiency in adults.

Autoantibodies directed against both the gastric parietal cells and IF are detectable in the serum and gastric juice of most patients. Damage to the parietal cells and failure of formation and absorption of the B_{12}–IF complex result. Achlorhydria is an accompanying feature (parietal cells are also responsible for secreting H^+).

Pernicious anaemia is associated with autoimmune thyroid disease, and patients are at increased risk of gastric carcinoma.

Clinical features include:
- A lemon-yellow colour to the skin, due to a combination of pallor and jaundice resulting from ineffective erythropoiesis.
- Glossitis.
- Gastrointestinal disturbances.
- Weight loss.
- Neurological abnormalities (peripheral neuropathy, subacute degeneration of the cord involving the posterior and lateral columns).
- Psychiatric disturbances.

The diagnosis is made using the **Schilling test**, the steps of which are as follows:

1. Oral, radioactively labelled B_{12} and intramuscular, non-radioactive B_{12} are administered simultaneously. The intramuscular B_{12} saturates the B_{12}-binding proteins in the plasma, thus promoting urinary excretion of any absorbed radioactive B_{12}.

2. The urine is collected for 24 hours after B_{12} administration and its radioactivity levels are measured. If less than 10% of the orally administered B_{12} is excreted, absorption of B_{12} is considered impaired.

3. The test is repeated, but this time both oral IF and oral B_{12} are given. If impaired absorption is due to lack of IF (as in pernicious anaemia), B_{12} absorption will be increased. If, however, malabsorption is the cause of B_{12} deficiency, B_{12} absorption will not be increased upon repeating the test.

Treatment of vitamin B_{12} deficiency is by correction of the underlying cause, if possible, and intramuscular injections of vitamin B_{12}.

Folate deficiency

The parent form of folate is pteroyl glutamic acid. Folate is found in foods of animal and plant origin and is destroyed by cooking. Absorption takes place in the duodenum and jejunum. Folate is stored in the liver. In contrast to the situation with vitamin B_{12}, stores are smaller and daily losses are larger relative to daily requirement, therefore a megaloblastic anaemia develops a few months after the onset of folate deficiency.

Causes of folate deficiency are:
- Decreased intake, e.g. due to poor diet.
- Decreased absorption, e.g. due to coeliac disease.
- Increased requirement due to rapid cell multiplication, e.g. caused by malignancy.
- Increased loss, e.g. due to desquamation.
- Drugs, e.g. methotrexate.

Clinical features of folate deficiency are similar to those of vitamin B_{12} deficiency, with the exception of the neurological and psychiatric abnormalities. Treatment of folate deficiency is by correction of the underlying cause, if possible, and giving oral supplements of folic acid.

Anaemia of chronic disease

Anaemia of chronic disease results from impaired red cell production. It is possibly due to a defect in the transfer of iron from the bone marrow macrophages to the red cell precursors.

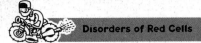

It is associated with:
- Chronic infections such as tuberculosis and osteomyelitis.
- Chronic diseases such as rheumatoid arthritis and SLE.
- Malignancies.

Haematological findings include:
- Normocytic, normochromic, or microcytic, hypochromic anaemia.
- Reduced serum iron and TIBC.
- Normal or high serum ferritin.
- Normal or low serum transferrin.
- Normal or increased bone marrow iron stores.

The last three findings distinguish the microcytic, hypochromic type from iron-deficiency anaemia. The anaemia does not respond to iron therapy and is correctable only by treatment of the underlying cause.

Aplastic anaemia

Aplastic anaemia is characterized by a pancytopenia (i.e. a reduction in all three cell lines—red cells, neutrophils, and platelets) and aplasia (hypocellularity) of the bone marrow. There is a reduction in the number of bone marrow stem cells and those that remain are defective and cannot repopulate the marrow. Causes of aplastic anaemia are listed in Fig. 14.7.

Other causes of marrow failure
Pure red cell aplasia
This disorder is a rare condition, where only the red cell precursors in the bone marrow are defective. White cell and platelet counts are normal.

Myelophthisic anaemia
This disorder is caused by space-occupying lesions, e.g. metastatic carcinoma in the bone marrow, which destroy bone marrow architecture.

Chronic renal failure
This disorder is almost always associated with anaemia. A decreased renal mass results in reduced production of erythropoietin (see p. 64).

Causes of aplastic anaemia	
Congenital	**Acquired**
Fanconi's anaemia—a rare, autosomal recessive condition associated with other congenital anomalies and an increased incidence of malignancy	idiopathic (50% of cases probably due to immune mechanisms)
	drugs—idiosyncratic reaction (e.g. chloramphenicol) or predictable, dose-related reaction (e.g. busulphan)
	chemicals, e.g. benzene
	irradiation
	infections, e.g. hepatitis C

Fig. 14.7 Causes of aplastic anaemia.

- Summarize the causes, clinical features, and laboratory findings of iron-deficiency anaemia.
- Summarize the causes, clinical features, and laboratory findings of meglaoblastic anaemias.
- What are the features of anaemia of chronic disease?
- What is aplastic anaemia? List some causes.

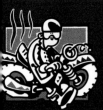

15. Disorders of Haemostasis

Definitions

The following definitions are useful here:

- Haemorrhage—loss of blood from the circulation.
- Petechiae—tiny punctate haemorrhages, less than 2 mm in diameter, usually occurring in clusters.
- Ecchymoses—diffuse flat haemorrhages under the skin. These are larger than petechiae and are commonly known as bruises.
- Purpura—this term includes both petechiae and ecchymoses and is used to describe any condition where there is bleeding into the skin or mucous membranes.
- Haematoma—loss of blood involving the subcutaneous tissue or muscle and resulting in a distinct localized swelling.

Bleeding disorders may be associated with a reduced platelet count (thrombocytopenia) or defects in platelet function.

Thrombocytopenia (reduced platelet count)

Decreased platelet production

This is the commonest cause of thrombocytopenia. The reasons for decreased platelet production are listed in Fig. 15.1.

Generalized disease of the bone marrow

Decreased megakaryocyte production, and consequently decreased platelet production, may be part of a wider clinical picture seen in aplastic anaemia, leukaemia, the myelodysplastic syndromes, and myelofibrosis. These are all diseases associated with generalized bone marrow failure. Bone marrow infiltration due to metastatic carcinoma, multiple myeloma, and lymphoma, also reduces the number of marrow megakaryocytes.

Specific impairment of platelet production

Drugs suppress platelet production by impairing megakaryocyte development. In certain cases, the production of drug-dependent antiplatelet antibodies also occurs. Ethanol also suppresses megakaryocyte proliferation and may be associated with mild platelet dysfunction: thrombocytopenia is a common complication in patients with alcoholism. Chemotherapy and radiotherapy both cause marrow depression,

Causes of decreased production of platelets	
Mechanism	**Cause**
bone marrow failure	aplastic anaemia
bone marrow infiltrate	metastatic carcinoma
	leukaemia
	myelofibrosis
	multiple myeloma
	lymphoma
impairment of platelet production	thiazides
	co-trimoxazole
	phenylbutazone
	alcohol
	chemotherapy or radiotherapy
	viruses, e.g. measles, HIV
ineffective megakaryopoiesis	megaloblastic anaemia
	amegakaryocytic thrombocytopenia
	paroxysmal nocturnal haemoglobinuria (PNH)

Fig. 15.1 Causes of decreased production of platelets.

reducing the number of haematopoietic cells including megakaryocytes. Viruses such as measles impair platelet production by invading the megakaryocyte. Approximately 50% of HIV patients develop thrombocytopenia due to the development of antiplatelet antibodies and HIV-induced suppression of megakaryocytes.

Ineffective megakaryopoiesis

Impaired DNA synthesis in megaloblastic anaemia due to vitamin B_{12} or folate deficiency results in ineffective thrombopoiesis. Amegakaryocytic thrombocytopenia is a rare disorder characterized by isolated thrombocytopenia secondary to decreased platelet production in the bone marrow. Other causes include paroxysmal nocturnal haemoglobinuria (PNH).

Decreased platelet survival

The causes of decreased platelet survival are listed in Fig. 15.2.

Causes of decreased platelet survival	
Mechanism	**Cause**
immune-mediated destruction	acute ITP
	chronic ITP
	neonatal alloimmune thrombocytopenia
	post-transfusion purpura
drug-induced ITP	quinine
	rifampicin
infections	bacterial sepsis, measles, rubella, influenza
	malaria
non-immune	thrombotic thrombocytopenic purpura
	dilutional thrombocytopenia
	splenomegaly
	DIC

Fig. 15.2 Causes of decreased survival of platelets.

Immune destruction

Acute idiopathic thrombocytopenic purpura (acute ITP) is a self-limiting illness that occurs most commonly in children under the age of 10 years. It follows viral infections of childhood such as rubella, chicken-pox, or measles. The platelet count is usually less than $20 \times 10^9/L$. The immune response to the virus leads to the circulation of antibody–viral antigen complexes, which bind onto the platelet surfaces and are subsequently removed by the reticuloendothelial system. Over 80% of patients recover without any treatment, but in 5–10% of cases, chronic idiopathic thrombocytopenic purpura (chronic ITP) develops.

Chronic idiopathic thrombocytopenic purpura occurs predominantly between the ages of 15 and 50 years. The incidence is greater in women than in men. Patients present with petechiae, ecchymoses, epistaxis, and menorrhagia. The platelet count is usually $20–80 \times 10^9/L$. Chronic ITP is usually idiopathic, but can also be seen in other disorders associated with aberrant immune responses, such as systemic lupus erythematosus (SLE). The onset is usually insidious and there is no history of a recent viral infection. Thrombocytopenia arises from the development of IgG autoantibodies to the platelet glycoproteins. The IgG–platelet complexes are removed by macrophages in the spleen. If platelets are coated with complement in addition to IgG, they are destroyed mainly in the liver. Chronic ITP rarely resolves spontaneously and the disease is characterized by episodes of remission and relapse.

Neonatal alloimmune thrombocytopenia is associated with the transfer of antiplatelet antibodies across the placenta, from the mother to the fetus.

Post-transfusion purpura occurs when thrombocytopenia develops 5–10 days after a transfusion because of antibody development against the antigen PI^{A1} found on the donor's platelets but not on the recipient's platelets. The reason for the destruction of the recipient's platelets is unclear.

Drug-induced immune thrombocytopenia

Certain drugs have been implicated in drug-induced immune thrombocytopenia (see Fig. 15.2). The platelet count is often less than $10 \times 10^9/L$ and patients present with acute purpura. A number of different mechanisms of platelet destruction have been proposed. This is an indication for cessation of drug therapy.

Non-immune destruction

Thrombotic thrombocytopenic purpura (TTP) is a rare but serious disorder that most commonly affects young adults. It is marked by fever, transient neurological defects, and renal failure. There is widespread deposition of 'platelet–fibrin' microthrombi in arterioles and capillaries, resulting in thrombocytopenia. Microangiopathic haemolytic anaemia is also a characteristic feature and arises from the fragmentation of erythrocytes as they circulate through the partially occluded vessels. The exact aetiology of TTP is unknown, but immune-mediated endothelial damage and synthesis of abnormal forms of von Willebrand's factor (vWF) causing platelet hyperaggregatability have been proposed as possible contributory factors.

Haemolytic–uraemic syndrome (HUS) is a similar disorder affecting infants and young children. However, in HUS, the platelet–fibrin microthrombi are limited to the kidneys. In many patients, the disease follows recent infections with *E. coli* and other enteric pathogens.

Disseminated intravascular coagulation

See p. 159.

Splenic sequestration

In a normal individual, about 30% of total body platelets are in the spleen at any one time. These are freely exchangeable with those in the circulation. An increase in splenic size (splenomegaly) due to portal hypertension causes the splenic platelet pool to increase to the point that it may account for up to 90% of total body platelets, resulting in peripheral thrombocytopenia.

Dilutional thrombocytopenia

Whole blood that has been stored for more than 24 hours contains very few viable platelets, owing to their short half-life. Massive transfusion (>10 units/24 h) of this platelet-poor blood can result in dilutional thrombocytopenia and deficiency of clotting factors II, V, and VIII.

Defects of platelet function

These may be congenital or acquired (Fig. 15.3).

Causes of defective platelet function	
Disorder	**Cause**
congenital	defective adhesion: Bernard–Soulier syndrome
	defective aggregation: Glanzmann's thromboaesthenia
	defective secretion: storage pool diseases
acquired	aspirin therapy
	uraemia

Fig. 15.3 Causes of defective platelet function.

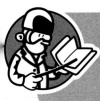

- Summarize the conditions in which bleeding occurs as a result of decreased platelet production and survival.
- List the congenital and acquired defects of platelet function that predispose to bleeding.

BLEEDING DISORDERS: CLOTTING FACTOR ABNORMALITIES

Clotting factor abnormalities may be hereditary or acquired.

Hereditary factor abnormalities

Von Willebrand's disease

This is the most common hereditary bleeding disorder, affecting 1% of the population. The most common form of the disease—von Willebrand type I—is characterized by a deficiency of circulating vWF, resulting from impaired release of normally synthesized vWF multimers from endothelial cells. vWF is the carrier protein for factor VIII in plasma, and stabilizes it, prolonging its survival in the circulation.

Type IIA von Willebrand's disease is caused by an absence of the largest vWF subunits. Type IIB von Willebrand's disease is due to the synthesis of abnormal vWF multimers by endothelial cells. The net result is a deficiency or defect of vWF. Clinical manifestations arise due to impairment of platelet adhesion to the subendothelium or due to a defect in the coagulation pathway caused by a factor VIII deficiency.

Haemophilia A and haemophilia B

Haemophilia A is caused by a deficiency of factor VIII, and haemophilia B (Christmas disease) by a deficiency of factor IX. Both are inherited as X-linked recessive disorders and therefore overwhelmingly affect males. The incidence of haemophilia A in males is 1 in 5000, representing a five times greater prevalence than for haemophilia B. In 33% of all haemophilia A cases, patients have no family history of the disease and such cases are thought to arise from spontaneous mutation of the gene responsible for factor VIII production. The normal plasma concentrations of factors VIII and IX range from 0.5 to 2 IU/mL. The frequency and severity of bleeding correlates with the level of factor VIII or IX in the patient: haemophilias A and B can be classified as severe, moderate, or mild (Fig. 15.4)

Other deficiencies

Hereditary deficiencies of the other coagulation factors are rare. As in haemophilias A and B, the severity of the disorders is related to the degree of deficiency.

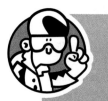

Haemophilias A and B are commonly examined topics. Know about the pattern of inheritance, pathophysiology, and clinical consequences.

Classification of haemophilia A and B		
Disease classification	**Level of coagulation factor VIII/IX (of normal)**	**Clinical manifestations**
severe	<2%	spontaneous haemorrhages into the joints (haemarthroses); recurrent bleeding can lead to joint destruction and crippling
moderate	2–5%	post-traumatic or post-surgical bleeding
mild	5–20%	post-traumatic bleeding

Fig. 15.4 Classification of haemophilias A and B.

Acquired factor abnormalities
Vitamin K deficiency
Vitamin K deficiency is discussed in Chapter 6.

Liver disease
The liver produces all the clotting factors except for vWF; liver disease is therefore associated with clotting factor deficiency. In addition, biliary obstruction can lead to malabsorption and deficiency of fat-soluble vitamin K. This leads to decreased synthesis of the vitamin-K-dependent factors II, VII, IX, and X by the liver. Portal hypertension may lead to splenomegaly, resulting in increased splenic sequestration of platelets. In severe liver disease, levels of factor V, and fibrinogen are reduced, and increased levels of plasminogen activator are present. An acquired dysfibrinogenaemia (functional abnormality of fibrinogen) is also seen in many patients.

Disseminated intravascular coagulation
Disseminated intravascular coagulation (DIC) arises from excessive activation of the intrinsic or extrinsic coagulation pathways, followed by activation of the fibrinolytic system. The coagulation pathways are activated in two ways:
- Release of tissue factor from damaged tissues, monocytes, or red blood cells.
- Activation of factors XII and XI by damaged vascular endothelium.

There is generalized fibrin deposition on vascular endothelium, with extensive consumption of platelets and coagulation factors. Fibrin deposition activates the fibrinolytic pathway and results in the formation of fibrin degradation products (FDPs).

FDPs inhibit fibrin polymerization and consequently impair coagulation. The net result is a bleeding disorder due to a lack of platelets and clotting factors and inhibition of fibrin polymerization by FDPs.

Causes of DIC include:
- Obstetric complications.
- Carcinoma.
- Infections.
- Trauma.
- Hypersensitivity.

○ **Summarize the various hereditary and acquired clotting factor abnormalities that result in bleeding.**

THROMBOSIS

Thrombosis is the formation of a semi-solid mass in the circulation from blood constituents during life. Virchow's triad outlines the factors that predispose to thrombus formation:
- Changes in blood flow.
- Changes in blood constituents.
- Changes within the walls of blood vessels.

Thrombophilia
Thrombophilias are disorders of haemostasis that increase the tendency of blood to clot. These may be inherited or acquired.

Primary (hereditary) thrombophilia
Antithrombin III deficiency
Inheritance of antithrombin III (ATIII) deficiency is autosomal dominant. The deficiency is either type I (decreased quantity) or type II (reduced biological activity). ATIII is usually activated by binding to endothelial-cell-associated heparin sulphate and inhibits thrombus formation on the endothelium. Affected individuals are usually heterozygous for this disorder and have 40–50% of normal plasma ATIII levels. Most patients with ATIII deficiency experience a thrombotic episode before the age of 50 years. Thrombosis may be severe and recurrent, and these patients may have to have their blood anticoagulated with oral warfarin (see also p. 83).

Deficiencies of proteins C and S

Inheritance for both protein C and protein S deficiencies is autosomal dominant. Diseases are either type I (decreased quantity) or type II (reduced biological activity). Heterozygotes have 50% of normal levels of proteins C or S, and clinical features are similar to ATIII deficiency. Homozygous individuals have less than 1% of normal levels of proteins C or S. Proteins C and S have a shorter half-life than vitamin-K-dependent factors II, IX, and X, and warfarin therapy, consequently results in a prothrombotic state for the first day, and may lead to skin necrosis. Protein S deficiency is clinically indistinguishable from protein C deficiency (see also p. 83).

Defective fibrinolysis

Rarely, abnormal plasminogen or fibrinogen have been associated with reduced fibrinolytic activity and a tendency of blood to clot.

Activated protein C deficiency

A mutation of the factor V gene (arginine is replaced by glutamine) renders factor V resistant to inactivation by activated protein C. This disorder has an incidence in Caucasians of 5% and it may account for the majority of cases of inherited thrombophilia.

Secondary (acquired) thrombophilia

The following conditions are associated with an increased incidence of thrombosis:

- Prolonged immobilization of the patient (venous stasis).
- Disseminated cancer (secretion of tumour substances that activate factor X).
- Oestrogen therapy (increased plasma levels of factors II, VII, IX, and X, and reduced levels of ATIII and tissue plasminogen activator).
- Myeloproliferative disorders.
- Sickle cell anaemia.
- The antiphospholipid antibody syndrome (lupus anticoagulant syndrome). This disorder is characterized by the presence of antiphospholipid antibodies. The main features of this syndrome are arterial and venous thrombosis in renal, cerebral, and mesenteric vessels. The disease may be idiopathic or secondary to other autoimmune disorders such as SLE.
- Factors such as smoking, hypercholesterolaemia, hypertension, infection, and immune-mediated damage, contribute to endothelial injury and subsequent thrombus formation.

- **What is Virchow's triad?**
- **List the hereditary and acquired conditions that predispose to thrombosis.**

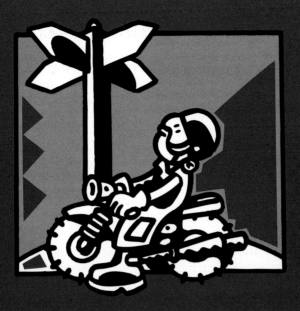

SELF-ASSESSMENT

Multiple-choice Questions   163

Short-answer Questions   168

Essay Questions   169

MCQ Answers   170

SAQ Answers   171

Multiple-choice Questions

Indicate whether each answer is true or false.

1. Concerning primary and secondary lymphoid tissue:

(a) The thymus is a secondary lymphoid organ.
(b) Lymph node follicles contain mainly T cells.
(c) The periarteriolar sheath in the white pulp of the spleen contains mainly T cells.
(d) Lymph nodes sample antigen from the blood.
(e) Peyer's patches are part of the diffuse mucosal-associated lymphoid tissue.

2. Regarding hypersensitivity reactions:

(a) Type I hypersensitivity reactions are mediated by IgG.
(b) Type III hypersensitivity involves the formation of immune complexes.
(c) Mast cells play a key role in immediate hypersensitivity.
(d) Delayed-type hypersensitivity mechanisms play a key role in haemolytic disease of the newborn due to Rhesus incompatibility.
(e) The Arthus reaction is a localized type III reaction.

3. Concerning acute inflammation:

(a) Acute inflammation is characterized by infiltration of neutrophils and vascular changes.
(b) Histamine is an important mediator.
(c) The complement system does not play a role.
(d) The coagulation and fibrinolytic systems are activated.
(e) Downregulation of ICAM-1 and ICAM-2 occurs.

4. Concerning chronic inflammation:

(a) Chronic inflammation is always preceded by acute inflammation.
(b) The macrophage plays a central role.
(c) Granuloma formation is a characteristic feature.
(d) Tissue destruction and regeneration occur simultaneously.
(e) Lymphocytes are not usually present.

5. Platelets:

(a) Are derived from the cytoplasm of the megakaryocyte.
(b) Are nucleated.
(c) Contain ADP in their α granules.
(d) Promote wound healing.
(e) Bind to von Willebrand's factor on damaged endothelial cells.

6. Concerning the coagulation cascade:

(a) All coagulation factors are either proenzymes or cofactors.
(b) The intrinsic pathway is activated by tissue factor.
(c) Thrombin converts soluble fibrinogen to a stable form of fibrin.
(d) Factors II, VII, VIII, and IX are vitamin-K-dependent.
(e) The action of antithrombin III is enhanced by warfarin.

7. Live vaccines are used to prevent:

(a) Polio.
(b) Tetanus.
(c) Tuberculosis.
(d) Rubella.
(e) Hepatitis B.

8. Rheumatoid factor:

(a) Is found in all cases of rheumatoid arthritis.
(b) Is an autoantibody.
(c) Is directed against IgM.
(d) Can activate complement.
(e) Amplifies the inflammatory response.

9. Features of β-thalassaemia major include:

(a) A very unwell infant at birth.
(b) Hepatosplenomegaly.
(c) A microcytic, hypochromic anaemia.
(d) Bony abnormalities.
(e) Iron overload.

10. Concerning generation of antigen receptor diversity:

(a) Both the light and heavy immunoglobulin chain variable regions are encoded by V, D, and J gene segments.
(b) Diversity can only be generated before encountering antigen.
(c) In B cells, N-nucleotide addition occurs only in heavy chains.
(d) Somatic hypermutation occurs in both B and T cells.
(e) Antibodies produced late in an immune response have decreased affinity for antigen.

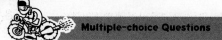

11. Erythrocytes:

(a) Have a diameter of 7–8 μm.
(b) Have multilobed nuclei.
(c) Are derived from pronormoblasts.
(d) Carry carbon dioxide primarily in the form of carbamino compounds.
(e) Have an average lifespan of 70 days.

12. Concerning iron metabolism:

(a) Iron is absorbed in the stomach.
(b) Iron is transported around the body in the form of ferritin.
(c) Most of the body's iron is found in stores in the liver, bone marrow, and spleen.
(d) Increased absorption can be compensated for by increased excretion.
(e) There is a failure of iron excretion in primary haemochromatosis.

13. Concerning haemoglobin:

(a) The principal haemoglobin in adults is HbA ($\alpha_2\beta_2$).
(b) Binding of oxygen to haemoglobin causes oxidation of the iron atom.
(c) The oxygen dissociation curve of haemoglobin is hyperbolic.
(d) The Bohr effect describes the shift of the oxygen dissociation curve with changes in pH.
(e) Increased 2,3-diphosphoglycerate (2,3-DPG) concentrations cause a shift of the oxygen dissociation curve to the left.

14. IgA:

(a) Is important in mucosal immunity.
(b) Is found in breast milk.
(c) Is the most abundant immunoglobulin in the blood.
(d) Crosses the placenta.
(e) Can fix complement.

15. Macrophages:

(a) Exhibit a more pronounced respiratory burst than neutrophils.
(b) Can present antigen to T cells.
(c) Have receptors for complement components.
(d) Are activated by IFN-γ.
(e) Are part of the mononuclear phagocyte system.

16. The following are features of iron-deficiency anaemia:

(a) Glossitis.
(b) Low serum ferritin.
(c) Koilonychia.
(d) Low total iron-binding capacity.
(e) Macrocytes.

17. Causes of absolute polycythaemia include:

(a) Polycythaemia rubra vera.
(b) Cyanotic heart disease.
(c) Hydronephrosis.
(d) Fluid depletion.
(e) Gaisbock's syndrome.

18. Warm autoimmune haemolytic anaemia is characterized by:

(a) The presence of IgG autoantibodies.
(b) Intravascular haemolysis.
(c) Worsening of symptoms in cold weather.
(d) A positive direct Coombs' test.
(e) Spherocytes.

19. The human leucocyte antigen (HLA) complex:

(a) Encodes major histocompatibilty complex (MHC) molecules.
(b) Is located on chromosome 16.
(c) Encodes some complement components.
(d) Has few alleles at each locus.
(e) Is a cluster of tightly linked genes.

20. Concerning class I MHC molecules:

(a) A class I molecule is made up of α- and β-chains.
(b) CD8+ T cells are class-I-MHC-restricted.
(c) Class I molecules are present only on antigen-presenting cells (APCs).
(d) Class I molecules present endogenous antigen.
(e) A class I molecule can bind longer peptides than a class II molecule because the peptide-binding cleft is more open.

21. The following are components of the innate immune system:

(a) Interferon.
(b) T cells.
(c) Complement.
(d) Antibody.
(e) Acute phase proteins.

22. Acute haemolytic transfusion reactions:

(a) Acute haemolytic transfusion reactions are caused by the destruction of donor red blood cells by antibodies present in the recipient's serum.
(b) Complement activation may occur.
(c) Symptoms develop within a few days.
(d) Hypertension, flushing, urtucaria, diarrhoea, and vomiting ensue.
(e) There is a danger of disseminated intravascular coagulation.

23. HLA matching is performed routinely before the transplantation of:

(a) Kidney.
(b) Heart.
(c) Skin.
(d) Bone marrow.
(e) Cornea.

24. Concerning kidney transplantation:

(a) If the donor and recipient are genetically identical at the HLA loci, a rejection response cannot occur.
(b) Hyperacute rejection occurs due to pre-existing antidonor antibodies.
(c) Acute cellular rejection occurs within minutes to hours.
(d) Antirejection therapy is required to prevent acute vascular rejection.
(e) Acute cellular rejection is mediated by T cells.

25. The following are examples of primary immunodeficiencies:

(a) Chronic granulomatous disease.
(b) Transient hypogammaglobulinaemia of infancy.
(c) Splenectomy.
(d) AIDS.
(e) Wiskott–Aldrich syndrome.

26. DiGeorge syndrome is characterized by:

(a) Damage to the third and fourth pharyngeal pouches.
(b) Thymic aplasia.
(c) Hyperparathyroidism.
(d) Cardiac defects.
(e) Recurrent infections.

27. Features of HIV infection include:

(a) Polyclonal B cell activation.
(b) Defective T cell function.
(c) A reversal of the CD4:CD8 ratio.

(d) Neutralizing antibodies directed against gp120 and gp41.
(e) Persistent generalized lymphadenopathy.

28. Amyloid deposition is associated with:

(a) Osteoarthritis.
(b) Familial Mediterranean fever.
(c) Dialysis.
(e) Medullary carcinoma of the thyroid.
(f) Alzheimer's disease.

29. Concerning Hodgkin's disease:

(a) It characteristically affects young females in the third and fourth decades of life.
(b) Diagnosis requires the presence of Reed–Sternberg cells.
(c) Disease severity is directly proportional to the number of lymphocytes in the lesion.
(d) Reed–Sternberg cells have a characteristic 'Orphan-Annie' appearance.
(e) Reed–Sternberg cells are thought to be the malignant cells of Hodgkin's disease.

30. Concerning acute lymphoblastic leukaemia (ALL):

(a) It accounts for 80% of all childhood leukaemias.
(b) Its peak incidence is at 12–15 years of age.
(c) It does not respond well to therapy and the remission rate is less than 50%.
(d) In 80% of cases, the blast cells are of B cell origin.
(e) The FAB classification divides ALL into three different groups on a morphological basis.

31. Concerning chronic lymphocytic leukaemia (CLL):

(a) It occurs most frequently in patients aged over 60 years.
(b) It accounts for 20% of all leukaemias.
(c) It arises from a neoplastic proliferation of B cells in approximately 95% of cases.
(d) Disease transformation to acute leukaemia does not occur.
(e) Median survival is 10–12 years.

32. Bleeding may occur as a consequence of:

(a) Drug therapy.
(b) Chemotherapy and radiotherapy.
(c) Blood transfusions.
(d) Splenomegaly.
(e) Defective platelet adhesion.

33. Regarding the complement system:

(a) Complement components are proteins or glycoproteins.
(b) Complement can only be activated by the alternative and classical pathways.
(c) The alternative pathway is usually activated by IgM and IgG.
(d) Complement components C5, C6, C7, C8, and C9 comprise the membrane-attack complex.
(e) The conversion of C3 to C3b by C3 convertase is the major amplification process in the complement cascade.

34. Concerning systemic lupus erythematosus (SLE):

(a) SLE is an organ-specific autoimmune disease.
(b) SLE is more common in men than in women.
(c) SLE is characterized by antinuclear autoantibodies.
(d) The presence of HLA-DR5 and HLA-DR6 haplotypes confers an increased risk of developing SLE.
(e) Exposure to infra-red rays results in an SLE-like disease.

35. Concerning rheumatoid arthritis (RA):

(a) RA is characterized by inflammation of the synovium and destruction of the articular cartilage.
(b) Approximately 30% of patients carry the HLA-DR1 and HLA-DR4 haplotypes.
(c) Rheumatoid factor is pathognomonic for RA.
(d) RA is more common in women than in men.
(e) Approximately 7% of the world's population suffers from RA.

36. The following autoimmune diseases are organ-specific:

(a) Reiter's syndrome.
(b) Hashimoto's thyroiditis.
(c) Myasthenia gravis.
(d) Graves' disease.
(e) Polyarteritis nodosa.

37. Hereditary spherocytosis is characterized by:

(a) An autosomal dominant pattern of inheritance.
(b) Intravascular haemolysis.
(c) The presence of spherocytes on the peripheral blood smear.
(d) Increased osmotic fragility of red cells.
(e) Decreased autohaemolysis of red cells.

38. Features of intravascular haemolysis include:

(a) Haemoglobinuria.
(b) Haemosiderinuria.
(c) Raised haptoglobulin levels.

(d) Increased red cell breakdown primarily in the bone marrow, liver, and spleen.
(e) Methaemalbuminaemia.

39. Glucose-6-phosphate dehydrogenase deficiency is characterized by:

(a) An autosomal recessive pattern of inheritance.
(b) The presence of Heinz bodies and bite cells on the peripheral blood smear.
(c) Invariably low levels of glucose-6-phosphate dehydrogenase during haemolytic crises.
(d) A severe African form of the disease.
(e) Protection of the heterozygous state from malaria caused by *Plasmodium falciparum*.

40. The following statements relate to the sickle syndromes:

(a) Sickle haemoglobin is characterized by a single base substitution of the β-chain gene.
(b) Deoxygenated sickle haemoglobin is more soluble than deoxygenated haemoglobin A.
(c) Sickle cell anaemia clinically manifests at about 6 months of age.
(d) Adults with sickle cell anaemia often have enlarged spleens.
(e) The sickling and solubility tests are negative in sickle cell trait.

41. Concerning recognition molecules of the immune system:

(a) Immunoglobulin molecules consist of two heavy chains and two light chains.
(b) The variable regions of the heavy and light chains are identical.
(c) The framework regions of immunoglobulins comprise the antigen-binding site.
(d) The T cell surface antigen receptor is a complex consisting of a T cell receptor associated with CD3.
(e) Approximately 95% of T cells express γδ receptors and the rest express αβ receptors.

42. Concerning plasma proteins:

(a) Albumin is essential for maintaining oncotic pressure and also acts as a transport molecule.
(b) Alpha-1-antitrypsin is a protease inhibitor and can have four different genetic variants: M, J, T, and Z.
(c) Homozygotes with the PiZZ genotype produce 60% of normal levels of α_1-antitrypsin.
(d) Caeruloplasmin is a carrier protein for zinc.

166

(e) High-density lipoprotein (HDL) is the major carrier of cholesterol.

---

43. Concerning the acute phase response:

(a) There is a change in the concentration of a number of plasma proteins.
(b) Leucocytosis and thombocytopenia develop.
(c) Levels of caeruloplasmin and α_1-glycoprotein undergo a 100–1000-fold increase.
(d) Levels of C-reactive protein and serum amyloid A rise within hours of tissue injury.
(e) The acute phase response is sustained even in the most severe illness.

---

44. Regarding red cell antigens:

(a) ABO antigen status is inherited and involves three allelic genes: A, B, and O.
(b) Both the A and B genes may be inherited, resulting in blood group AB.
(c) IgG antibodies usually develop in all immunocompetent humans against blood group antigens not present on their own cells.
(d) Approximately 85% of Caucasians are Rhesus-positive.
(e) Rhesus-negative persons generate antibody directed against Rhesus antigens because of exposure to naturally occurring D-antigen-like antigens in intestinal bacteria and food substances.

---

45. Self-tolerance may be due to:

(a) Early clonal deletion
(b) Clonal anergy.
(c) Molecular mimicry.
(d) Selective lymphocyte migration.
(e) T-cell mediated supression.

---

46. Leucocytosis may be associated with:

(a) Diabetic ketoacidosis.
(b) Uraemia.
(c) Psoriasis.
(d) Megaloblastic anaemia.
(e) Autoimmune disease.

---

47. In multiple myeloma:

(a) A malignant polyclonal proliferation of bone marrow plasma cells occurs.
(b) Terminal-deoxynucleotidyl-transferase-negative CD10+ lymphoid cells have been proposed as the original clonogenic cells.

(c) IgM is secreted more often than IgG by the malignant cells.
(d) A macrocytic anaemia may develop.
(e) Hypercalcaemia is a presenting feature in the majority of patients.

---

48. In Waldenström's macroglobulinaemia:

(a) A neoplastic proliferation of cells belonging to the B cell lineage occurs.
(b) The tumour cells are present in the bone marrow, blood, lymph nodes, and spleen.
(c) An IgG paraprotein is always secreted.
(d) Most patients present between the third and fifth decades of life.
(e) A bleeding tendency is often present.

---

49. Clotting factor abnormalities are found in:

(a) Von Willebrand's disease.
(b) Haemophilias A and B.
(c) Excess vitamin K.
(d) Vitamin C deficiency.
(e) Bernard–Soulier syndrome.

---

50. Causes of neutropenia include:

(a) Drug therapy.
(b) Aplastic anaemia.
(c) Leukaemias and lymphomas.
(d) Iron-deficiency anaemia.
(e) Hypersplenism.

167

Short-answer Questions

1. Explain what the HLA complex is and briefly mention its functions.

2. What is the Bohr effect? Use a sketch to illustrate your answer.

3. Describe what happens in a delayed-type hypersensitivity reaction. Give two examples of antigens that can induce such a reaction.

4. Draw and label a cross-section through a lymph node.

5. What are the differences between Th1 and Th2 cells?

6. Explain what the term 'positive and negative selection of T cells' means and state where these processes take place.

7. Draw the classical complement pathway and explain how it is activated.

8. List the clinical features of haemolytic anaemias and explain how they arise.

9. Draw the structure of an Ig molecule and list the functions of Igs.

10. Write short notes on pernicious anaemia.

11. What is haemolytic disease of the newborn and how may it be prevented?

12. Define the following terms: innate and adaptive immunity; antigen; immunogen; hapten; epitope.

13. What are the differences between active and passive immunization? Outline the advantages and disadvantages of each.

14. Write short notes on the role of vitamin K in coagulation.

15. Draw and label a diagram of a platelet.

16. Outline the immunopathogenesis of rheumatoid arthritis.

17. Draw the band pattern obtained on normal serum electrophoresis. Outline the changes found in cirrhosis and multiple myeloma.

18. What are the tests that can be used to investigate bleeding?

19. Write short notes on Hodgkin's disease.

20. Write short notes on antithrombin III deficiency.

Essay Questions

1. Describe the different mechanisms that operate to generate diversity of the B and T cell antigen receptors.

2. Write an essay on the red cell cytoskeleton. What happens if it is defective?

3. Relate the structure of the immunoglobulin molecule to its functions.

4. Write an essay on sickle cell anaemia, with special reference to the pathogenesis, clinical features, and laboratory findings.

5. Compare and contrast the processes of acute and chronic inflammation.

6. Describe the process by which blood is cross-matched prior to transfusion. What happens if an O-negative patient receives blood from an AB-positive patient?

7. Describe the mechanisms that usually protect an individual from autoimmunity and discuss how they may break down.

8. Describe the pathogenesis, clinical features, and laboratory findings of multiple myeloma.

9. How is coagulation regulated?

10. Describe the four patterns of graft rejection and discuss how they may be prevented.

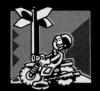

MCQ Answers

1. (a)F, (b)F, (c)T, (d)F, (e)F

2. (a)F, (b)T, (c)T, (d)F, (e)T

3. (a)T, (b)T, (c)F, (d)T, (e)F

4. (a)F, (b)T, (c)T, (d)T, (e)F

5. (a)T, (b)F, (c)T, (d)T, (e)T

6. (a)F, (b)F, (c)F, (d)F, (e)F

7. (a)T, (b)F, (c)T, (d)T, (e)F

8. (a)F, (b)T, (c)F, (d)T, (e)T

9. (a)F, (b)T, (c)T, (d)T, (e)T

10. (a)F, (b)F, (c)T, (d)F, (e)F

11. (a)T, (b)F, (c)T, (d)F, (e)F

12. (a)F, (b)F, (c)F, (d)F, (e)F

13. (a)T, (b)F, (c)F, (d)T, (e)F

14. (a)T, (b)T, (c)F, (d)F, (e)T

15. (a)F, (b)T, (c)T, (d)T, (e)T

16. (a)T, (b)T, (c)T, (d)F, (e)F

17. (a)T, (b)T, (c)T, (d)F, (e)F

18. (a)T, (b)F, (c)F, (d)T, (e)T

19. (a)T, (b)F, (c)T, (d)F, (e)T

20. (a)F, (b)T, (c)F, (d)T, (e)F

21. (a)T, (b)F, (c)T, (d)F, (e)T

22. (a)T, (b)T, (c)F, (d)F, (e)T

23. (a)T, (b)F, (c)F, (d)T, (e)F

24. (a)F, (b)T, (c)F, (d)F, (e)T

25. (a)T, (b)F, (c)F, (d)F, (e)T

26. (a)T, (b)T, (c)F, (d)T, (e)T

27. (a)T, (b)T, (c)T, (d)T, (e)T

28. (a)F, (b)T, (c)T, (d)T, (e)T

29. (a)F, (b)T, (c)F, (d)F, (e)T

30. (a)T, (b)F, (c)F, (d)T, (e)T

31. (a)T, (b)F, (c)T, (d)T, (e)F

32. (a)T, (b)T, (c)T, (d)T, (e)T

33. (a)T, (b)F, (c)F, (d)F, (e)T

34. (a)F, (b)F, (c)T, (d)F, (e)F

35. (a)T, (b)F, (c)F, (d)T, (e)F

36. (a)F, (b)T, (c)T, (d)T, (e)F

37. (a)T, (b)F, (c)T, (d)T, (e)F

38. (a)T, (b)T, (c)F, (d)F, (e)T

39. (a)F, (b)T, (c)F, (d)F, (e)T

40. (a)T, (b)F, (c)T, (d)F, (e)F

41. (a)T, (b)F, (c)F, (d)T, (e)F

42. (a)T, (b)F, (c)F, (d)F, (e)F

43. (a)T, (b)F, (c)F, (d)T, (e)T

44. (a)T, (b)T, (c)F, (d)T, (e)F

45. (a)T, (b)T, (c)F, (d)T, (e)T

46. (a)T, (b)T, (c)T, (d)F, (e)F

47. (a)F, (b)T, (c)F, (d)F, (e)F

48. (a)T, (b)T, (c)F, (d)F, (e)T

49. (a)T, (b)T, (c)F, (d)F, (e)F

50. (a)T, (b)T, (c)T, (d)F, (e)T

1. The HLA (human leucocyte antigen) complex is the human major histocompatibility complex (MHC) and is located on chromosome 6. The genes of the HLA complex are divided into the class I, II, and III regions, which are further subdivided into loci. There are a large number of alleles at each locus and the loci are tightly linked. Most individuals are heterozygous at each locus and the alleles are expressed codominantly. The class I region is divided into A, B, and C loci, and encodes the class I MHC molecules (present on virtually all of the nucleated cells of the body). The class II region is divided into DP, DQ, and DR loci, and encodes the class II MHC molecules (present primarily on antigen-presenting cells).

   The class I and class II molecules present processed antigen to CD8+ and CD4+ T cells, respectively. They are important in the rejection of transplanted tissues.

   The molecules encoded by the class III region include complement components and tumour necrosis factor (TNF).

2. The Bohr effect describes the shift of the oxygen dissociation curve for haemoglobin to the right in response to increased hydrogen ion concentration. A modified form of Fig. 5.10 can be used to illustrate this.

3. Delayed-type (type IV) hypersensitivity is the body's response to certain antigenic stimuli. It can be divided into a sensitization and an effector phase. The sensitization phase lasts 1–2 weeks: upon first exposure to antigen, a subset of CD4+ T helper (Th) cells is clonally expanded. Upon subsequent exposure, the sensitized Th cells secrete cytokines that attract and activate macrophages (the effector phase). The cytokines secreted include interleukin-2 (IL-2), interferon-γ (IFN-γ), and TNF-β. IL-2 autoactivates the Th cells so that they produce more cytokines. IFN-γ and TNF-β are chemotactic for monocytes and macrophages and facilitate their extravasation. In addition, IFN-γ activates macrophages so that they are more efficient at presenting antigen (thus activating more T cells) and have increased lytic and phagocytic ability (so that they can destroy pathogens more effectively). The macrophages are the main effector cells in type IV reactions. It takes 48–72 hours to reach the peak of the effector phase: this time is required for the recruitment and activation of macrophages.

   Delayed-type hypersensitivity reactions can result from infection with *Mycobacterium tuberculosis* and contact with nickel.

4. Refer to Fig. 2.2.

5. Refer to Fig. 3.26.

6. Positive and negative selection of T cells occurs during T cell maturation in the thymus. Positive selection of T cells refers to the process whereby T cells that are capable of binding self-MHC molecules are selected for. It involves the interaction of the developing CD4+ CD8+ T cells with thymic epithelial cells that express high levels of class I and class II MHC molecules. T cells that do not interact with MHC are presumed to undergo apoptosis as they do not receive a protective signal as a result of the interaction between the T cell receptor (TCR) and MHC. Some of the T cells that survive positive selection have high affinity for MHC. These CD4+ CD8+ T cells undergo negative selection. Negative selection is thought to be mediated by dendritic cells and macrophages (both of which are derived from the bone marrow). These cells express high levels of class I and II MHC molecules, which interact with T cells expressing high-affinity receptors for self-MHC alone or self-MHC and antigen. These 'self-reactive' T cells are, therefore, removed via apoptosis.

   Positive and negative selection results in T cells that moderately recognize foreign antigens in conjunction with self-MHC molecules. Positive selection occurs in the cortex of the thymus. Negative selection occurs in the corticomedullary junction and medulla of the thymus.

7. A modified form of Fig. 3.30 can be used to illustrate the classical pathway. The classical pathway can be activated by immune complexes containing IgG and IgM. The CH2 domain (IgG) or the CH3 domain (IgM) binds the C1q component. IgM is much more effective than IgG at activating complement.

8. The information in Fig. 5.7 is required here.

9. Fig. 3.9 shows the structure of an Ig molecule. The functions are as follows:
   - Complement fixation.
   - Opsonization.
   - Neutralization of toxins.
   - Participation in antibody-dependent cell-mediated cytotoxicity.
   - Protection of the neonate (transplacental passage).

10. Pernicious anaemia is a chronic atrophic gastritis with a probable autoimmune aetiology. It is the commonest cause of vitamin B_{12} deficiency in adults. Autoantibodies directed against both the gastric parietal cells and intrinsic factor (IF) are detectable in the serum and gastric juice of most patients. Damage to the parietal cells and failure of formation and absorption of the B_{12}–IF complex result.

Achlorhydria is an accompanying feature (parietal cells are also responsible for secreting H^+). Pernicious anaemia is associated with autoimmune thyroid disease and patients are at increased risk of gastric carcinoma. Clinical features include:

- A lemon-yellow colour to the skin, caused by a combination of pallor and jaundice resulting from ineffective erythropoiesis.
- Glossitis.
- Gastrointestinal disturbances.
- Weight loss.
- Neurological abnormalities (peripheral neuropathy, subacute degeneration of the spinal cord involving the posterior and lateral columns, psychiatric disturbances <aq4>).

The diagnosis is made using the Schilling test.

11. Haemolytic disease of the newborn can result when the fetus of a Rhesus-negative mother is Rhesus-positive. The mother is usually sensitized at birth, when small amounts of fetal blood leak into the maternal circulation. The mother mounts an antibody response directed against the Rhesus antigens; so, during subsequent pregnancies where the fetus is Rhesus-positive, IgG antibodies cross the placenta and bind to fetal red cells, resulting in haemolysis. Most cases are due to anti-D antibodies. The most severe consequence is hydrops fetalis.

Prevention is by intramuscular administration of anti-D IgG to the Rhesus-negative mother at 28 weeks and within 72 hours after birth. The D surface antigen on fetal red blood cells in the maternal circulation is coated, thereby preventing a maternal immune response. The Rhesus-positive red blood cell–anti-D antibody complex is then removed in the maternal reticuloendothelial system (RES).

12. Innate immunity comprises the non-specific mechanisms that exist prior to exposure to antigen and are not altered on repeated exposure to a particular antigen.

Adaptive immunity is characterized by specificity and memory. Specificity refers to the ability of the adaptive immune response to distinguish minor differences between antigens. Memory refers to the fact that once the adaptive immune system has responded to an antigen, it responds more rapidly and to a greater degree upon subsequent exposures.

An antigen is any molecule that can be recognized by the adaptive immune system.

An immunogen is a molecule that evokes an immune response. All immunogens are antigenic, but not all antigens are immunogenic.

A hapten is a small antigen that is not immunogenic unless coupled to a larger (usually protein) carrier molecule.

An epitope (antigenic determinant or immunologically active portion of antigen) is the discrete area of the antigen which is recognized by the adaptive immune response.

13. Fig. 4.10 can be used to answer this question.

14. Factors II, VII, IX, and X, and proteins C and S are dependent on vitamin K for post-translational modification (see Fig. 6.7).

Vitamin K acts as a cofactor for the carboxylase enzyme, resulting in γ-carboxylation of glutamic acid residues, enabling them to bind calcium and, therefore, form complexes with the platelet phospholipid membrane.

In the absence of vitamin K, factors II, VII, IX, and X—termed 'proteins induced by vitamin K absence' (PIVKA)—do not undergo γ-carboxylation, cannot bind calcium, and are unable to attach onto platelet phospholipid membranes. Consequently, they are activated much more slowly and negligible levels of prothrombin are converted into thrombin.

15. Fig. 6.1 can be used to answer this question.

16. Fig. 12.2 can be used to answer this question.

17. Fig. 7.1 can be used to answer the first part of this question.

In cirrhosis, there is a decrease in albumin and a diffuse increase in γ-globulins, resulting in βγ fusion. In multiple myeloma, a distinct band appears in the γ-globulin region owing to the production of paraprotein.

18. A good way to answer this question is to draw out the algorithm in Fig. 9.5. It saves time and simplifies the answer.

19. Hodgkin's disease (HD) characteristically affects young males in the third and fourth decades of life. Diagnosis requires the presence of the Reed–Sternberg (RS) cell or one of its derivatives in all cases. These pathognomonic cells are typically mixed with a variable inflammatory infiltrate.

Disease severity is directly proportional to the number of RS cells found in the lesions and is indirectly linked to the numbers of lymphocytes in the lesions. The

RS cell and its variants have been proposed at the malignant cells of HD.

RS cells are binucleated or multinucleated, with prominent eosinophilic nucleoli, giving rise to the so-called owl's-eye appearance.

Variants of RS cells are lacunar cells and the uninucleated, polylobated RS cell.

The REAL classification divides HD into five histological subtypes:

- Lymphocyte predominance—this accounts for 10% of cases of HD and has a good prognosis.
- Mixed cellularity—this accounts for 30% of cases of HD.
- Lymphocyte depletion—this accounts for 10% of cases of HD and has the poorest prognosis among all forms of HD.
- Nodular sclerosis—this accounts for 50% of cases of HD and, unlike the other forms, is found more frequently in women.
- Lymphocyte-rich classic HD (provisional entity).

Although histological composition is an important prognostic factor in HD, clinical staging (Ann-Arbor staging) is the most accurate indicator of long-term prognosis.

20. Antithrombin III (ATIII) is a naturally occurring inhibitor protein that binds to activated clotting factors, especially thrombin, and inactivates them. It also inhibits factors XIIa, XIa, Xa, IXa, and VIIa.

ATIII is usually activated by binding to endothelial-cell-associated heparin sulphate and inhibits thrombus formation on the endothelium. ATIII deficiency is either type I (decreased quantity) or type II (reduced quality, i.e. reduced biological activity). Inheritance is autosomal dominant. Affected individuals are usually heterozygous for this disorder and have 40–50% of normal plasma ATIII levels. By the age of 50 years, most patients with ATIII deficiency have had a thrombosis, which may be severe and recurrent, and these patients may be anticoagulated with oral warfarin.

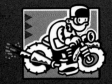

Index

A

abdomen, examination, 103, 104
abdominal lymph nodes, 10
ABO antigens, 89
achlorhydria, 153
acquired immunodeficiency syndrome *see* AIDS
acrocyanosis, 150
actin (band 5), 73
activated partial thromboplastin time (APTT), 83
activated protein C, 83, 160
   deficiency, 160
acute phase proteins, 87
acute phase response, 87
adjuvants, 56
ADP, 78, 79
adventitial reticular cells, 7
affinity maturation, 33
agammaglobulinaemia, 125
agglutination, 25
agranulocytosis, 133
AIDS, 126–9
   see also HIV/HIV infection
AIDS-related complex (ARC), 128
albumin, 85
alcoholism, 155
alleles, 27
allelic exclusion, 31
allergens, 49
allergic disorders, 49
allergic responses, 19, 49
allogeneic graft, 58
allotype, 25
alpha-1 antitrypsin, 85–6
   alleles, 85
   deficiency, 86
alpha-1-globulins, 85
alpha-2-antiplasmin, 84
alpha-2-globulins, 86
alpha-2-macroglobulin, 84, 86
Alzheimer's disease, 131
amylin, 131
amyloid, 130
   AA type, 130, 131
   of ageing (senile cardiac), 131
   AL (light chain) proteins, 130, 131
   β-amyloid (A4 protein), 131

serum amyloid A (SAA), 87, 130
amyloidosis, 130–1
   dialysis-associated, 130
   hereditary, 131
   localized, 130, 131
   primary, 130, 140
   reactive systemic (secondary), 130
   systemic, 130–1
anaemia, 97, 145
   aplastic, 108, 133, 154
   blood loss causing, 145
   causes, 145
   of chronic disease, 64, 153–4
   diagnostic algorithm, 98
   differential diagnoses, 97
   Fanconi's, 154
   haemolytic *see* haemolytic anaemia
   in impaired red cell production, 152–4
   iron-deficiency *see* iron-deficiency anaemia
   macrocytic, 152
   Mediterranean (Cooley's), 147
   megaloblastic, 108, 133, 152–3
   microcytic hypochromic, 148, 152, 154
   myelophthisic, 154
   pernicious, 54, 125, 153
   recombinant erythropoietin use, 64
   red cell destruction causing *see* haemolytic anaemia
   refractory, 139
   refractory with excess blasts (RAEB), 139
   sickle cell *see* sickle cell anaemia
   sideroblastic, 139
   signs/symptoms, 152
anaphylatoxins, 52
anaphylaxis, 49
anergy, T cell, 53
anisocytosis, 107
ankylosing spondylitis, 55
ankyrin, 72, 73
antibiotics, 17
antibodies, 33
   affinity maturation, 33
   calculation of diversity, 32
   diversity, 30–3
   hypersensitivity mechanisms, 49
   immunity mediated by *see* humoral immunity
   neutralizing, 25, 33, 53, 128

antibodies *continued*
    primary/secondary responses, 15, 16
    to receptors, 49
    see also autoantibodies; immunoglobulin(s)
antibody-dependent cell-mediated cytotoxicity (ADCC), 25, 33, 49, 52
anti-DNA antibodies, 121
anti-D (RhD) antibodies, 90
antigen, 15, 33
    binding, Fab fragment role, 22
    clearance mechanisms, 33
    graft/transplantation, 58
    persistence, 45, 48
    presentation to T cells, 29–30
    processing, 28–9, 34
    sequestered, release, 54
    T cell dependent, 34
    T cell independent, 33
antigenic determinant (epitope), 15, 22, 25
antigenic shift/drift, 53
antigen-presenting cells (APCs), 5, 11, 21, 28, 29, 34
antiphospholipid antibody syndrome, 160
α_2-antiplasmin, 84
antirejection therapy, 59
antithrombin III (ATIII), 83, 159
    deficiency, 149
antitoxins, 56
α_1-antitrypsin *see* alpha-1 antitrypsin
aplastic anaemia, 108, 133, 154
apoptosis, 9, 35
arachidonic acid, 44
arms, examination, 102
Arthus reaction, 50–1
asplenia, congenital, 143
atopy, 49
ATP, 73
Auer rods, 107, 137
auscultation, 101
autoantibodies, 111, 121
    in pernicious anaemia, 153
autoantigens, 54
autohaemolysis, 146
autoimmune disease, 54–5, 121–4
    aetiologies, 55
    haemolytic anaemias, 50, 106, 150, 151
    organ-specific, 122–4, 125
    pathogenic mechanisms, 54, 122
    systemic, 121–2, 123
autoimmunity, 53–5
autologous graft, 58
axillary lymph nodes, 9
azathioprine, 59
azurophilic granules, 18, 114

B
bacille Calmette–Guérin (BCG) vaccination, 51
bacteria
    immune response, 52
    molecular mimicry, 54
bacteria infections, passive immunization, 56
band 3 protein, 72
band 4.1 protein, 73
basophilic stippling, 148
basophils, 19, 20
    functions, 5, 19
    increased count, 135
    normal appearance, 114
    normal range, 106
    structure, 18, 114
B cell(s), 4, 22–6
    antibody diversity, 30–3
    antigenic specificity, 26
    counts, 111
    in lymph node cortex, 10
    maturation, 7, 26, 30
    polyclonal activation, 54, 128
    recognition molecules, 22–6
    self-tolerance, 53
    surface antigen receptor (membrane Ig), 4, 25–6, 30
    surface markers (CD19/CD20), 111
    see also antibodies; immunoglobulin(s)
B cell leukaemia, 138
B cell lymphomas, 136, 137
Bence Jones protein, 116, 130, 139
Bernard-Soulier syndrome, 157
β cells, 54, 124
beta-globulins, 86
bicarbonate, 62
biopsy
    lymph node, 109, 117
    trephine, of bone marrow, 105, 117
'bite' cells, 147
blast cells, leukaemia, 107, 137
blast crisis, 138
bleeding disorders, 97, 155–7
    clotting factor abnormalities, 158–9
    defective platelet function, 157
    diagnostic algorithm, 99
    differential diagnoses, 98
    thrombocytopenia-associated, 155–7
bleeding time, 83
'blister' cells, 147
blood
    carbon dioxide carriage, 62
    cross-matching, 91, 106
    loss, 145, 155
    oxygen carriage, 61

blood *continued*
  storage, 82
blood cells, 3, 4
  functions, 5
  normal/abnormal, imaging, 112–16
  see also red blood cells; white blood cells
blood donors, universal, 89
blood films, peripheral, 112
  abnormal, 105, 107, 115–16
  normal, 112–14
blood products, 92
blood sinusoids, 7
blood supply, spleen, 12
blood transfusions, 89, 91–2
  ABO compatible, 89
  ABO incompatible, 50, 89, 91
  acute haemolytic reactions, 91
  autologous, 64
  cross-matching, 91, 106
  dilutional thrombocytopenia, 157
  emergency, 92
  iron overload, 66
  thrombocytopenia and purpura after, 156
Bohr effect, 71
bone marrow, 4, 7
  abnormal appearance, 108
  aplasia, 154
  aspiration and biopsy, 105, 117
  depression, 155–6
  erythropoiesis, 63
  examination, 105, 117
  failure, 154, 155
  fibrosis (myelofibrosis), 142
  infiltrates, 155
  normal appearance, 117
  red and yellow types, 7
  see also myelodysplastic syndromes
bradykinin, 44, 46
bruises (ecchymoses), 155
Bruton, X-linked agammaglobulinaemia, 125
Burkitt's lymphoma, 109
burns, immunodeficiency in, 126
bursa of Fabricius, 7

C

C1 inhibitor, 41, 127
caeruloplasmin, 86, 87
calcitonin, 131
calcium, role in coagulation, 82
cancer
  amyloidosis associated, 131
  disseminated, thrombophilia in, 160
carbamino compounds, 62

carbon dioxide
  carriage in blood, 62
  haemoglobin curve and, 70, 71
CD3 antigen, 26, 27
CD4 antigen, 30
CD4$^+$ T cells, 28, 29, 30, 36, 37
  in bacterial infections, 52
  counts, 112
  in HIV infection and AIDS, 127, 128
  MHC restriction, 29, 30
  in protozoan infections, 53
  in viral infections, 52
  see also T cell(s), helper (Th)
CD8 antigen, 30
CD8$^+$ T cells, 28, 29, 30, 37
  in bacterial infections, 52
  counts, 112
  MHC restriction, 29, 30
  in protozoan infections, 53
  in viral infections, 52
CD40 and CD40L, 34
cell adhesion molecules (CAMs), 43
cell lineages, 3
cell-mediated immunity, 35–8
  to bacteria, 52
  deficiency, 124, 126
  phases, 51
  to protozoa, 53
  tests, 112
  type IV hypersensitivity, 51
  to viruses, 52
  see also T cell(s)
cervical lymph nodes, 9
chemotactic agents, 44
chemotaxis, 44
chloramines, 19
chloride shift, 62
Christmas disease (haemophilia B), 92, 158
chronic granulomatous disease, 127
cirrhosis, 86
  primary biliary, 125
clinical examination, 101–4
clonal anergy, 53
clonal deletion, 53
clotting factors *see* coagulation factors
coagulation, 44, 80–4
  activation, 44, 80
  cascade and components of, 80–4
  defects, 83
  disseminated intravascular (DIC), 91, 159
  excessive activation, 159
  extrinsic pathway, 81
  inhibitors, 82, 83

coagulation *continued*
  intrinsic pathway, 80, 81
  platelet plug and, 79, 80
  regulatory pathways, 83–4
  vitamin K and calcium role, 82
coagulation factors, 80, 82, 92
  abnormalities, 158–9
  concentrates, 92
  see also specific factors
co-factors, 80
cold autoimmune haemolytic anaemia, 150, 151
collagen, synthesis, chronic inflammation, 47
colony-forming unit (CFU), 4
colony-stimulating factors (CFSs), 4, 78
complement, 17, 38–41, 86
  activation, 25, 38–9, 49, 91
  activation by bacteria, 33, 52
  activation by immunoglobulins, 25, 33
  alternative pathway, 25, 38–9
  amplification, 40
  C3b, 38, 39, 52
  CH_{50} screen, 110
  classical pathway, 25, 38, 39
  common terminal pathway, 39–40
  components, 38
  deficiencies, 110, 126, 127
  fixation, 54
  function, 40
  function tests, 110
  inhibitors, 40, 41, 110, 150
  lectin pathway, 38, 39
  membrane-attack complex (MAC), 40, 52
  regulators of complement activation (RCA), 41
complementarity-determining regions (CDRs), 24, 27
Cooley's anaemia, 147
Coombs' test, 106, 108, 150
C-reactive protein, 17, 87
cross-matching, blood, 91, 106
cryoprecipitate, 92
cyclosporin, 59
cytogenetic analysis, 109
cytokines, 4, 15
  in bacterial infections, 52
  humoral immune response, 34
  imbalance, 54
  in inflammation, 44
  receptors, 4
  released by Th1/Th2 cells, 36
  see also erythropoietin; specific interleukins
cytotoxicity, antibody-dependent cell-mediated (ADCC),
  25, 33, 49, 52
cytotoxic T cells, 37

D

decay-accelerating factor (DAF), 41, 150
defensins, 19
degranulation, 19, 25
  tests, 111
delayed-type (type IV) hypersensitivity, 48, 51, 54
deoxyhaemoglobin, 70
desferrioxamine, 66
diabetes mellitus
  insulin-dependent, 54, 124
  insulin-resistant, 131
dialysis-associated amyloidosis, 130
diapedesis, 44
DiGeorge syndrome (thymic aplasia), 9, 126
2,3-diphosphoglycerate, 70, 71, 73
direct antiglobulin (Coombs') test, 106, 108, 150
disseminated intravascular coagulation (DIC), 91, 159
domains, 23
Donath–Landsteiner antibodies, 150
drug history, 96
drugs
  immune haemolytic anaemia due to, 161
  immune thrombocytopenia due to, 157
  neutropenia due to, 133–4
  platelet production decreased by, 155
dysfibrinogenaemia, 159

E

ecchymoses (bruises), 155
electrophoresis
  haemoglobin, 106, 109
  serum *see* serum electrophoresis
ELISA (enzyme-linked immunosorbent assay), 110, 128
elliptocytosis, hereditary, 146
Embden–Meyerhoff pathway (glycolytic), 73, 75
embryology, thymus development, 9
emphysema, panacinar, 86
endomitosis, 77
endothelial cells, 7, 63
eosinophilic granuloma, 140
eosinophils, 19
  development, 19
  functions, 5
  increased counts, 135
  normal appearance, 113
  normal range (count), 106
  structure, 18, 113
epithelioid cells, 48
epitope (antigenic determinant), 15, 22, 25
erythrocytes, 5, 61–2, 63
  see also red blood cells
erythrocyte sedimentation rate (ESR), 87
erythroid hyperplasia, 66

erythroid progenitor cells, 3, 63
erythropoiesis, 63–4, 146
    compensatory, 68
    ineffective, 63, 152
    regulation, 63–4, 67
    sequence, 63
erythropoietin (EPO), 4, 63–4, 67
    decreased production, 63–4, 154
    inappropriate sensitivity, 142
    recombinant, 64
Evan's syndrome, 150
examination, clinical, 101–4

F

Fab fragments, 22
FAB (French–American–British) classification, leukaemia,
    137, 138
factor V, 83, 160
factor VIIa, 80, 81
factor VIII, 80
    deficiency, 158
factor IX, deficiency, 158
factor Xa, 79, 80
factor XI, 80
factor XII (Hageman factor), 44, 80
factor XIII (fibrin-stabilizing factor), 80
factor B, 39
factor D, 39
factor H, 39, 41
factor I, 41
familial amyloid polyneuropathy, 131
familial Mediterranean fever, 131
family history, 96
Fanconi's anaemia, 154
Farmer's lung, 51
favism, 147
Fc fragment, 22
Felty's syndrome, 143
ferritin, 7, 66
fibrin, 44, 80
    degradation, 44, 83, 84, 159
    generalized deposition, 159
fibrin degradation products (FDPs), 44, 83, 84, 159
fibrinogen, 44, 80, 87
    deficiency/abnormal, 83
    elevated, 87
fibrinolysis, 44, 83–4
    defective, 160
    intrinsic/extrinsic activators, 83
fibrinopeptides, 44
fibroblasts, 7
    migration, chronic inflammation, 47
folate deficiency, 153

N-formylmethionine, 44
fragments X and Y, 84
fresh frozen plasma (FFP), 92

G

gamma-globulins, 86
    see also immunoglobulin(s)
Ganzmann's thromboasthenia, 157
gastritis, chronic atrophic, 153
gastrointestinal tract, lymphoid tissues, 13
Gaucher's disease, 143
germinal centers, 12
giant cells, multinucleate, 48
globin chains, 69, 71
    in sickle cell anaemia, 148, 149
    in thalassaemia, 147, 148
    see also haemoglobin
globin genes, 71
glossitis, 152, 153
glucose, red cell metabolism, 73–6
glucose-6-phosphate dehydrogenase (G6PD) deficiency,
    74, 76, 146–7
glutathionine (GSH), 74
glycolytic pathway (Embden–Meyerhoff), 73, 75
glycophorins, 72
glycoproteins, platelet, 78
    GPIIb/IIIa, 78, 79
glycosyl-phosphatidylinositol (GPI), 150
Goodpasture's syndrome, 125
grafts see transplantation
granulocyte(s), 17–19
    accelerated removal, 133
    destruction, 133, 134
    structure, 18
    see also basophils; eosinophils; neutrophils
granulocyte colony-stimulating factor (G-CFS), 4
granulocyte–macrophage colony-stimulating factor
    (GM-CSF), 4, 78
granulocytopenia see neutropenia
granuloma, formation, 48
granulopoiesis, inadequate, 133
Graves' disease, 49, 55, 123

H

haem, 66–8, 68, 69
haemagglutination tests, 111
haematological investigations, 105–9, 112–16
haematoma, 155
haemochromatosis, 66, 86
haemoglobin, 61, 68–71
    adult (HbA), 69
    Barts, 148
    defects, 147–50

haemoglobin *continued*
    degradation, 67
    electrophoresis, 106, 109
    fetal (HbF), 69, 148
    Gower, 69
    haem pocket, 69, 70
    H (HbH) disease, 148
    low levels, in anaemia, 145, 152
    normal range, 105
    physiological properties, 70–1
    Portland, 69
    S (HbS), 148
    structure, 68–70
    types, 69
    see also anaemia; globin chains
haemoglobinaemia, 146
haemoglobinuria, 146, 150
    paroxysmal nocturnal, 150
haemolysis, 91, 146
    extravascular, 91, 146
    in G6PD deficiency, 74, 76
    intravascular, 91, 146, 147
haemolytic anaemia, 67, 73, 145, 146–51
    acquired disorders, 145, 150–1
    alloimmune, 106, 161
    autoimmune, 50, 106, 150, 151
    bone marrow appearance, 108
    chronic, 149
    clinical features, 68
    Coombs' test in, 106
    drug-induced immune, 106, 161
    hereditary disorders, 73, 145, 146–50
    microangiopathic, 157
    non-immune, 161
haemolytic disease of newborn, 50, 90, 91, 151
haemolytic-uraemic syndrome (HUS), 157
haemophilia A and B, 92, 158
haemopoiesis, 3, 7, 63, 141
    ineffective (dysplastic), 138
    sites, 4, 7
    stages, 3
    see also erythropoiesis
haemopoietic stem cells, 3
    neoplastic proliferation *see* leukaemia
haemorrhage, 155
haemosiderin, 7, 66
haemosiderinuria, 146
haemosiderosis, 66
haemostasis, 77–84
    disorders, 155–60
    see also coagulation; platelet(s)
Hageman factor (factor XII), 44, 80
'hair-on-end' appearance, 118, 148

hands, examination, 102
Hand-Schüller-Christian disease, 140
haplotype, 27
hapten, 15
haptoglobulin, 86
    absence, 146
Hashimoto's thyroiditis, 54, 122–3
Hassall's corpuscles, 9
head, examination, 102, 103
Heinz bodies, 107, 147
heparin, 83
    low-molecular-weight, 83
hepatitis, neonatal, 86
hepatitis A, 57
hepatitis B, 57
herd immunity, 56
hereditary ataxia telangiectasia, 126
hereditary elliptocytosis, 146
hereditary spherocytosis, 73, 74, 115, 146
hereditary thrombophilia, 159–60
hexose monophosphate shunt, 74, 76
high endothelial venules (HEVs), 11
high-molecular-weight kininogen (HMWK), 44, 80
histamine, 44
histiocytosis X (Langerhans' cell histiocytosis), 140
history, presenting, 95
history-taking, 95–7
    history of presenting complaint, 95
    review of systems, 96
HIV/HIV infection, 126–9, 156
    immunology and laboratory features, 128–9
    structure (HIV-1), 126, 128
    transmission, 127
HLA (human leucocyte antigen), 27
    disease associations, 55, 121, 122, 123
    see also major histocompatibility complex (MHC)
Hodgkin's disease, 109, 117, 134
    classification, 136
    staging, 136
homologous restriction factor, 41, 150
Howell–Jolly bodies, 107
human immunodeficiency virus (HIV)
    see HIV/HIV infection
human leucocyte antigen *see* HLA
humoral immunity, 33–4
    to bacteria, 52
    deficiency, 124, 125
    to protozoa, 53
    tests, 111
    in viral infections, 52
    see also antibodies; B cell(s); immunoglobulin(s)
hydrogen peroxide, 19
hydrops fetalis, 90, 148

hydroxyl radical, 19
hyperacute rejection, 58
hypercalcaemia, 140
hypergammaglobulinaemia, 86
hypermutation, somatic, 33
hypersensitivity, 49–51
    type I (immediate), 19, 49
    type II (antibody-mediated), 49–50, 54
    type III (immune complex-mediated), 50–1, 54
    type IV (cell-mediated; delayed-type), 48, 51, 54
hypersplenism, 133, 143
hypochlorous acid, 19
hypochromia, 107
hypogammaglobulinaemia, 86, 125
    common variable, 125
    transient of infancy, 126
hypoxia, 63, 71

I

idiopathic thrombocytopenic purpura (ITP), 156
idiotope, 25
idiotype, 25
immune complexes
    circulation, 51
    formation, 50
    localized deposition, 50–1
    type III hypersensitivity, 50–1
immune response, 33–4
    evasion, 53
    to pathogens, 51–3
    primary/secondary, 15, 16
    to tissue damage, 43–9
    see also cell-mediated immunity; humoral immunity
immune system, 3–5
    adaptive, 15, 16, 52, 53
    cells, 16, 17–21, 22, 26
    components, 16
    disorders, 121–31
    innate, 15, 16, 16–21
    to pathogens, 51–2, 52, 53
    investigations, 110–12
immunity, 15–41
    adaptive, 15
    herd, 56
    innate *see* immune system, innate
    mucosal, 33
    see also cell-mediated immunity; humoral immunity
immunization, 55–7
    active, 55–6
    passive, 55, 56–7
    schedule (UK), 57
immunodeficiency disorders, 124–9
    primary, 124–6

secondary, 126–9
    severe combined (SCID), 126
    see also hypogammaglobulinaemia
immunogen, 15
immunoglobulin(s), 22
    antigen-binding site, 24
    classes, 22, 25
    class switching, 31–2
    constant domains, 24
    constant regions, 22
    domains, 23, 24
    fold structure, 23
    gene rearrangements, 30, 31, 32
    gene segments, 30
    gene superfamily, 26
    heavy chain, 22, 23
    heavy chain gene segments, 30, 31, 32
    hinge region, 24
    human normal, 57
    hypervariable regions, 24
    kappa light chains, 22, 31
    lambda light chains, 22
    light chain, 22, 23
    light chain gene segments, 30, 31
    membrane (mIg; B cell antigen receptor), 4, 25–6, 30
    monoclonal, 116, 139
    in passive immunization, 56, 57
    properties, 24
    secreted (sIg), 25, 26
    structure, 22–3
    structure-function relationship, 24
    variable domains, 23, 24
    variable regions, 22
    see also antibodies; specific immunoglobulins
immunoglobulin A (IgA), 13
    dimers, 25
    properties, 24
    selective deficiency, 125
    in viral infections, 52
immunoglobulin D (IgD), 24
immunoglobulin E (IgE), 24
    type I hypersensitivity, 49
immunoglobulin G (IgG), 24
    autoantibodies, 150, 156
    placental transfer, 126
    structure, 22
    subclasses, 24
immunoglobulin M (IgM), 24
    paraproteins, 140
immunological memory, 15
infants, transient hypogammaglobulinaemia, 126
infections
    decreased platelet survival, 156

infections *continued*
   repeated, 125, 127, 140
   splenomegaly, 143
inferior mesenteric lymph nodes, 10
inflammation, 43–9
   acute, 43–4, 46
   cells involved, 43, 45
   chronic, 45–8, 123
   in disease, 48
   results/effects of, 44, 45, 46
   vascular changes, 43, 45
inflammatory cells, 43, 45
inflammatory exudate, 43
inflammatory mediators, 44, 46
   formation and action, 45
inguinal lymph nodes, 10
inspection, 101
integrin family, 43
integrins, neutrophil expression, 44
interdigitating (ID) cells, 8
interferons, 17
   IFN-γ, 48, 51
   in viral infections, 51
interleukin, 4
interleukin-2 (IL-2), 21, 53
interleukin-3 (IL-3), 78
interleukin-8 (IL-8), 44
interleukin-10 (IL-10), 53
interstitial fluid, 9
intrinsic factor, 152
   antibodies, 54
investigations, 105–18
iron
   increased absorption, 66
   metabolism, uptake and excretion, 65–6
   overload, 65–6
   parenteral administration, 66
   storage, 7, 65
iron-deficiency anaemia, 108, 115, 152
   signs/symptoms, 152
isotypes, 25

J
J-chains, 25, 30
jugular venous pressure (JVP), 102

K
kallikrein, 80
killing of cells *see* lysis/killing of cells
kininogen, high-molecular-weight (HMWK), 44, 80
kinin system, 44
Kleihauer technique, 90
Kupffer cells, 21, 63

L
lactoferrin, 17, 19
lamina propria, 13
Langerhans' cell, 21, 140
Langerhans' cell histiocytosis (histiocytosis X), 140
large granular lymphocytes *see* natural killer (NK) cells
left shift, myeloid cells, 107, 116
Letterer-Siwe disease, 140
leucocyte adhesion deficiency, 127
leucocytes *see* white blood cells
leucocytosis, 134
leucoerythroblastic changes, 107
leucopenia, 133–4
leukaemia, 137–8
   acute lymphoblastic (ALL), 138
   acute myeloblastic (AML), 107, 137
   bone marrow appearance, 108
   chronic lymphocytic (CLL), 107, 108, 138
   chronic myeloid (granulocytic) (CML), 109, 110, 138
   chronic myelomonocytic (CMML), 139
   classification, 137, 138
   white cell abnormalities on blood film, 107
leukotrienes, 44
liver, palpation and percussion, 103
liver disease, clotting factor deficiency, 159
low-density lipoprotein (LDL), 86
lower limbs, examination, 102, 103
Luebering–Rapoport shunt, 73–4, 76
lupus anticoagulant syndrome, 160
lymph, 9
   flow in lymph nodes, 11
lymphatic drainage, 9–11
   function, 9
lymphatic vessels, 9, 10
   afferent and efferent, 11
lymph node, 9–11
   biopsy, 109, 117
   function, 9
   lymphatic flow in, 11
   structure, 10–11
lymphocytes, 4
   in chronic inflammation, 48
   functions, 5
   increased counts, 135
   large granular *see* natural killer (NK) cells
   normal appearance, 114
   normal range (count), 106
   recirculation, 11
   selective migration, tolerance due to, 53
   in spleen, 12, 13
   trafficking in MALT, 13
   see also B cell(s); T cell(s)
lymphoid cells, 3, 4

lymphoid organs/tissues, 7–13
    mucosal associated (MALT), 9, 13
    organization, 7–13
    primary, 7–13–9
    secondary, 9–13
    spleen *see* spleen
lymphokine-activated killer (LAK) cells, 21
lymphoma, 134, 136
    Burkitt's, 109
    classification, 134, 136, 137
    follicle-centre, 109
    Hodgkin's *see* Hodgkin's disease
    non-Hodgkin's, 136, 137
lymphopenia, 133, 134
lymphovenous junctions, 10
lysis/killing of cells
    complement mechanism, 40
    by cytotoxic T cells, 37
    in phagocytosis, 19
lysozyme, 17, 19

M
α_2-macroglobulin, 84, 86
macroglobulins, and macroglobulinaemia, 140
macrophage, 7, 21
    activated, 21, 47
    activation in type IV hypersensitivity, 51
    in chronic inflammation, 45, 47, 49
    epithelioid and giant cell formation, 48
    in liver (Kupffer cells), 21, 63
    neutrophil comparison, 21
    phagocytosis, 21
    receptors, 21
    secretory products, 21, 47
    in skin (Langerhans' cell), 21, 140
    splenic, 13
    structure and function, 21
macrophage colony-stimulating factor (M-CFS), 4
major histocompatibility complex (MHC), 26, 27–8
    antigen processing/presentation, 28–30
    class I molecules, 28
    class II molecules, 21, 28
    class III molecules, 27, 28
    genes, 27
    graft rejection, 58
    inappropriate expression, 54
    restriction, 30, 35
    self-MHC molecules, 30, 35
    structure and function, 28
    upregulation by interferon, 51
    see also HLA (human leucocyte antigen)
malabsorption, 126
malaria, 51, 150

malignancy *see* cancer
malnutrition, 126
mannan-binding protein (MBP), 38
margination, of neutrophils, 43–4
mast cells, 20
    degranulation, 25, 44
    mediators and actions of, 20, 44
M cells, 13
mean cell haemoglobin (MCH), 105
mean cell haemoglobin concentration (MCHC), 105
mean cell volume (MCV), 105
measles, 57
medical history, 96
Mediterranean (Cooley's) anaemia, 147
megakaryocytes, 77–8
    decreased production, 155
megakaryopoiesis, ineffective, 156
megaloblast, 152
megaloblastic anaemia, 108, 133, 152–3
membrane-attack complex (MAC), 40, 52
memory, immunological, 15
metachromasia, 18
methaemalbuminaemia, 146
microflora, skin and mucosal membranes, 17
β_2-microglobulin, 130
migration inhibition factor (MIF), 47
mitogen responses, T cells, 112
mixed connective tissue disease (MCTD), 123
molecular mimicry, 54
monoclonal gammopathy of undetermined significance
  (MGUS), 140
monocytes, 21
    functions, 5
    increased counts, 135
    normal appearance, 114
    normal range (count), 106
    see also macrophage
mononuclear phagocytic system, 21
mucosal associated lymphoid tissue (MALT), 9, 13
mucosal membranes, innate defence system, 17
multiple myeloma, 139–40
    amyloidosis in, 130, 140
    bone marrow appearance, 108
    peripheral blood film, 116
    skull radiograph, 120
myasthenia gravis, 49, 125
myelodysplastic syndromes, 138–9
myelofibrosis, 108, 142
myeloid stem cells, 3, 4
    differentiation pathways, 3, 141
    left shift, 107, 116
    neoplastic proliferation, 138, 140
myeloma

myeloma *continued*
    multiple *see* multiple myeloma
    solitary (plasmacytoma), 140
myeloma cells, 139
myeloperoxidase, 19
myeloproliferative disorders, 140–2
myoglobin, 70

N
NADPH, 74
natural killer (NK) cells, 4, 20–1
    killing mechanism, 21
    in viral infections, 51, 52
neck, examination, 102, 103
neonate *see* newborn
nephrotic syndrome, 86, 126
neutralization
    by antibodies, 25, 33, 53, 128
    of bacterial toxins and viruses, 33, 40
neutropenia, 127, 133, 139
    drug-induced, 133–4
neutrophilia, 135
neutrophils, 17, 19
    in acute inflammation, 43–4, 49
    chemotaxis, 44
    degranulation tests, 111
    destruction, 134
    diapedesis, 44
    extravasation, 43–4
    functions, 5, 17
    granules, 18, 19
    hypersegmentation, 107, 152
    increased counts, 135
    ineffective production, 133
    integrin expression, 44
    leucocytosis (neutrophilia), 135
    margination, 43–4
    normal appearance, 113
    normal range (count), 106
    phagocytosis by, 17, 19, 44
    production/differentiation, 19
    reduced count, 133–4
    structure, 18, 113
newborn
    RhD haemolytic disease, 50, 90, 91, 151
    transplacental passage of IgG, 25
Niemann–Pick disease, 143
nitroblue tetrazolium (NBT) reduction test, 111
nodular sclerosis, 136
non-Hodgkin's lymphoma, 136, 137
normoblasts, 63
nucleotides, in antibody diversity generation, 33
'nurse' cells, 8

O
oestrogen, 160
oncotic pressure, 85
opsonins, 21, 52
opsonization, 25, 40, 54
orchitis, autoimmune, 125
osteoclast-activating factor (OAF), 139
oxygen
    carriage in blood, 61–2
    dissociation curve, 70
    in haemoglobin, 70
    phagocytosis killing mechanism, 19

P
packed cell volume (PCV), 105, 140
pain, 95
palpation, 101
pancytopenia, 154
pannus, 121
paraproteins, 85, 139
    IgM, 140
parietal cells, autoantibodies, 153
paroxysmal cold haemoglobinuria, 150
paroxysmal nocturnal haemoglobinuria, 150
Paterson–Kelly syndrome, 152
pentose phosphate (hexose monophosphate) pathway, 74, 76
percussion, 101
periarteriolar lymphoid sheath (PALS), 12
pernicious anaemia, 54, 125, 153
petechiae, 155
Peyer's patches, 13
phagocytic cells, 17, 19, 21
    function tests, 111
    see also macrophage; neutrophils
phagocytosis, 7, 44
    deficiencies, 126, 127
    by eosinophils, 19
    by macrophage, 21
    by neutrophils, 17, 19
    oxygen-dependent degradation, 19
    oxygen-independent degradation, 19
phagolysosome, 53
phagosome, 19
Philadelphia chromosome, 109, 138
pigeon-fancier's disease, 51
plasma, 85
    fresh frozen (FFP), 92
    volume, 145
plasma cells, 22, 34
    in chronic inflammation, 48
plasmacytoma (solitary myeloma), 140
plasmin, 44, 83, 84

plasmin *continued*
  inhibitors, 84
plasminogen, 83, 84
plasminogen activators, 44, 83, 84
  inhibitors, 84
platelet(s), 77–9
  adhesion and aggregation, 78–9
  decreased production, 155–6
  decreased survival, 156–7
  defective function, 157
  disorders, 155–7
  elevated count, 106, 142
  functions, 5, 78–9
  granules, 77
  IgG autoantibodies, 156
  immune destruction, 156–7
  non-immune destruction, 157
  normal appearance, 112
  normal range (count), 106
  plug, 79, 80
  production, 77–8
  reduced count *see* thrombocytopenia
  splenic sequestration, 157
  storage and transfusion, 92
  structure, 77
platelet-activating factor (PAF), 44, 45
platelet-derived growth factor (PDGF), 47, 79
`platelet–fibrin' microthrombi, 157
Plummer–Vinson syndrome, 152
pluripotent stem cells, 3
pneumococcal vaccine, 146, 149
poikilocytosis, 107
polyarteritis nodosa (PAN), 123
polychromasia (reticulocytosis), 107, 145, 146, 147
polycythaemia, 140–2
  absolute, 140, 141
  apparent, 140, 141
polycythaemia rubra vera, 108, 142
polymorphism, 27
polymorphonuclear cells, 17
  see also granulocyte(s); neutrophils
polyneuropathy, familial amyloid, 131
porphyrins, 66
portal hypertension, 143
post-transfusion purpura, 156
presenting complaints, 97–9
  history of, 95
primary biliary cirrhosis, 125
proenzymes, 80
progenitor cells, 3, 4
pronormoblasts, 63
prostacyclin, 79
prostaglandins, 44, 77

protease inhibitor, 85
protein C, 82, 83
  activated, 83, 160
  deficiency, 160
protein S, 82, 83
  deficiency, 160
proteins induced by vitamin K absence (PIVKA), 82
prothrombin time, 83
protozoa, immune response, 52–3
pure red cell aplasia, 154
purified protein derivative (PPD), 51
purpura, 155
  idiopathic thrombocytopenic (ITP), 156
  post-transfusion, 156
  thrombotic thrombocytopenic (TTP), 157
pus, 17

R
rabies, 56
radiological investigations, 118
reactive lysis, 40
REAL classification, lymphoid neoplasms, 134, 136, 137
reciprocal proteolytic activation, 80
rectal examination, 103
red blood cells, 63
  abnormal counts, 105
  abnormalities on blood films, 107
  antibodies, 89, 90, 91, 106
  antigens, 89–91
  cytoskeleton, 72–3
  destruction, 146
  disorders, 145–54
  functions, 5, 61–2
  impaired production, 145, 152–4
  increased destruction, 145, 146–51
  lifespan, 61
  maturation, 63
  membrane defects, 146, 150
  metabolic defects, 73, 146–7
  metabolism, 73–6
  normal appearance, 112
  normal counts, 105
  osmotic fragility (increased), 146
  rouleaux, 87, 107, 116
  sickled, 107, 116, 148
  structure, 61, 63
  trauma, 161
  see also reticulocytes
Reed–Sternberg cells, 109, 117, 134, 136
Reiter's syndrome, 123
renal disease, decreased erythropoietin in, 63
renal failure, chronic, 140, 154
respiratory burst, 19

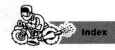

respiratory tract, lymphoid tissues, 13
reticulin fibres, 7
reticulocytes, 63
　count, 105, 113
　normal appearance, 113
reticulocytosis (polychromasia), 107, 145, 146, 147
reticuloendothelial system (RES), 90
RhD haemolytic disease of newborn, 50, 90, 91, 151
Rhesus antigens, 89–90
Rhesus disease, 50, 90, 91, 151
rheumatoid arthritis, 55, 121–2
　immunopathogenesis, 121, 122
Romanowsky-stain, 61, 63, 112
rouleaux, 87, 107, 116

S

Schilling test, 153
sebaceous glands, 17
selectin family, 43
self-tolerance, 53
　breakdown, 54–5
　mechanisms, 53–4
serology, 89–92
serum, 85
serum amyloid A (SAA), 87, 130
serum electrophoresis, 85
　abnormal, 86
　multiple myeloma, 139
serum proteins, 85–7
　normal, 85–6
serum sickness, 51
severe combined immunodeficiency disease (SCID), 126
sickle cell, 107, 116, 148
sickle cell anaemia, 71, 116, 149
　clinical features, 149
sickle cell β-thalassaemia, 150
sickle cell haemoglobin C disease, 150
sickle cell syndromes, 148–50
sickle cell trait, 150
sickling test, 149
sideroblast, 139
sideroblastic anaemia, 139
signal transduction, 27, 30
Sjögren's syndrome, 123
skin, innate defence system, 17
skin-prick test, 49
skin tests, 51, 112
skull radiographs, 118
smear cells, 107
social history, 96
somatic hypermutation, 33
spectrin, 73
　deficiency, 73, 74, 146

spherocytes, 107, 146
spherocytosis, hereditary, 73, 74, 115, 146
spleen, 12–13
　blood supply, 12
　congenital abnormalities, 143
　disorders, 143–4
　infarction, 143
　organization, 12
　platelet sequestration, 157
　red and white pulp, 12
　rupture, 143
splenomegaly, 143, 157
　congestive, 143
stem cell factor (SCF), 4
stem cells, 3, 7
　neoplastic proliferation, 137, 140
stromal cells, 8
subcapsular sinus, 11
superantigens, 38
superior mesenteric lymph nodes, 10
superoxide radical, 19
syngeneic graft, 58
systemic lupus erythematosus (SLE), 51, 121
systemic sclerosis, 123

T

tactoids, 148
target cells, 107, 116
T cell(s), 4
　activation, 53, 54
　antigen recognition, 26
　CD4+ see CD4+ T cells; T cell(s), helper (Th)
　CD8+ see CD8+ T cells
　clonal deletion and clonal anergy, 53
　cytotoxic killing mechanisms, 37
　cytotoxic (Tc), 37
　in graft rejection, 58, 59
　helper (Th), 11, 33, 34, 36, 51
　　functions, 36
　　subsets, 36
　　in viral infections, 52
　　see also CD4+ T cells
　inappropriate activation, 54
　in lymph node paracortex, 11
　maturation, 7, 8–9, 35
　MHC restriction, 30, 35
　positive/negative selection, 35
　recognition molecules, 26–30
　self-reactive, 35
　suppression, tolerance in, 53
　suppressor, 37
　surface antigen receptor, 26–7
T cell neoplasms, 136, 137

T cell receptor (TCR), 4, 26–7
  αβ and γδ types, 27
  antigen-binding cleft, 28, 38
  diversity and generation, 33
  downregulation, 53
  structure, 27
  superantigen binding, 38
teardrop cells, 107
telangiectasia, hereditary ataxia, 126
tetanus toxoid, 56
thalassaemia, 147–8
α-thalassaemia, 147
  syndromes, 148
β-thalassaemia, 71
  sickle cell, 150
  syndromes, 147, 148
β-thalassaemia major, 118, 147, 148
thorax, examination, 103, 104
thrombin, 44, 79, 80
thrombin time, 83
thrombocythaemia, primary, 106, 142
thrombocytopenia, 106, 139, 155
  amegakaryocytic, 156
  decreased platelet production, 155–6
  decreased platelet survival, 156–7
  dilutional, 157
  drug-induced immune, 157
  essential, 108
  idiopathic thrombocytopenic purpura, 156
  neonatal alloimmune, 156
  thrombotic thrombocytopenic purpura, 157
thrombocytosis, 106
thrombophilia, 159–60
  primary (hereditary), 159–60
  secondary (acquired), 160
thrombopoietin, 78
thrombosis, 159–60
thrombotic thrombocytopenic purpura (TTP), 157
thromboxane A$_2$, 79
thymic aplasia (DiGeorge syndrome), 9, 126
thymic epithelial cells, 8
thymocytes, 7, 8
thymus, 7–9
  development/embryology, 9
  size, 9
  T cell development, 35
  timescale of cell development, 9
  ultrastructure, 8
thyroid carcinoma, medullary, 131
thyroid disease, autoimmune, 54, 122–3, 153
thyroiditis, Hashimoto's, 54, 122–3
tissue damage, immune response, 43–9
tissue factor (factor III), 81

tissue matching, 59
tissue plasminogen activator (tPA), 44, 83
tissue repair, platelets role, 79
tonsils, 13
trabeculae, 8, 12
transferrin, 65, 86
transplantation, 58–9
  antigens, 58
  rejection, 58–9
  rejection prevention strategies, 59
  types/organs, 59
transthyretin, 131
trephine biopsy, 105, 117
trypanosomes, 53
tuberculin skin test, 51
tumour necrosis factor α (TNF-α), 44

U
ulcerative colitis, 125
urokinase plasminogen activator (uPA), 84

V
vaccination, 55
vaccines
  ideal, 55
  live vs killed, 57
  types, 56
varicella zoster, 57
vascular changes, in acute inflammation, 43, 45
vasodilatation, 43
venous stasis, 160
Virchow's triad, 159
viruses, 54
  immune response to, 51–2
  molecular mimicry, 54
  neutralization, 33, 40
virus infections, passive immunization, 56–7
vitamin B$_{12}$ deficiency, 152–3
vitamin K, 82
  deficiency, 82, 159
von Willebrand's disease, 158
von Willebrand's factor (vWF), 78, 80, 157, 158

W
Waldenström's macroglobulinaemia, 130, 140
warfarin, 82, 159
warm autoimmune haemolytic anaemia, 150, 151
wheal-and-flare reaction, 49
white blood cells
  abnormalities, 106, 107
  disorders, 133–44
  extravasation, 43–4
  neoplastic proliferation, 134–43

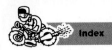

white blood cells *continued*
  normal count, 106
  raised counts, 134, 135
  reactive proliferation, 134, 135
  reduced count (leucopenia), 133–4
  structure and functions, 17–21
  see also individual cell types
Wiskott–Aldrich syndrome, 126

X

xenogeneic graft, 58
X-linked agammaglobulinaemia of Bruton, 125